Study Guide to Accompany

Foundations of Clinical Drug Therapy

Anne Collins Abrams, RN, MSN
Associate Professor, Emeritus
Department of Baccalaureate
   and Graduate Nursing
College of Health Studies
Eastern Kentucky University
Richmond, Kentucky

Sandra Smith Pennington, RN, PhD
Associate Professor of Nursing
Berea College
Berea Kentucky

and

Graduate Program Director
DSc Program in Nursing
Rocky Mountain University of Health Professions
Provo, Utah

Mary Jo Kirkpatrick, RN, MSN
Assistant Professor and Director
Associate of Science in Nursing
Mississippi University for Women
Columbus, Mississippi

D1455853

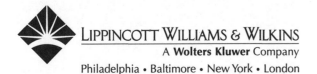
LIPPINCOTT WILLIAMS & WILKINS
A **Wolters Kluwer** Company
Philadelphia • Baltimore • New York • London
Buenos Aires • Hong Kong • Sydney • Tokyo

Managing Editor: Doris Wray
Director of Nursing Production: Helen Ewan
Managing Editor / Production: Erika Kors
Art Director: Carolyn O'Brien
Design Coordinator: Brett MacNaughton
Senior Manufacturing Manager: William Alberti
Compositor: Lippincott Williams & Wilkins
Printer: Victor Graphics

Eighth Edition

9 8 7 6 5 4 3 2 1

ISBN: 0-7817-5354-6

Care has been taken to confirm the accuracy of the information presented and to describe generally accepted practices. However, the authors, editors, and publisher are not responsible for errors or omissions or for any consequences from application of the information in this book and make no warranty, express or implied, with respect to the content of the publication.

The authors, editors, and publisher have exerted every effort to ensure that drug selection and dosage set forth in this text are in accordance with the current recommendations and practice at the time of publication. However, in view of ongoing research, changes in government regulations, and the constant flow of information relating to drug therapy and drug reactions, the reader is urged to check the package insert for each drug for any change in indications and dosage and for added warnings and precautions. This is particularly important when the recommended agent is a new or infrequently employed drug.

Some drugs and medical devices presented in this publication have Food and Drug Administration (FDA) clearance for limited use in restricted research settings. It is the responsibility of the health care provider to ascertain the FDA status of each drug or device planned for use in his or her clinical practice.

LWW.com

Contents

Preface

The *Study Guide to Accompany Foundations of Clinical Drug Therapy* has been developed to complement the text. It provides a wealth of learning opportunities to reinforce content that you have read in the text and to promote your ability to apply this information.

Pharmacology is a tough and demanding science, fraught with seemingly limitless detail about an ever-growing number of drugs. Helping students learn the principles of pharmacology as applied to nursing practice to foster safe and effective management of drug therapy is perhaps one of the most challenging tasks surrounding nursing education today.

This *Study Guide* offers a variety of activities that incorporate approaches to learning designed to accommodate many learning styles and increase the appeal of nursing. These exercises have been chosen to help you establish a connection between how a drug works and why it is used for a particular disorder.

Although each exercise is aimed at expanding your knowledge base and understanding of drug therapy, it also increases your understanding of what patients need to know to maximize client drug therapy. They also help you expand your personal knowledge of drug therapy, and help to develop critical thinking and test-taking skills. You will receive additional reinforcement from answers provided in the back of the workbook, which allow immediate feedback about the preciseness of exercise answers.

We hope that this *Study Guide* will be a very useful tool in helping you adapt and apply the basic concepts of clinical drug therapy.

Lippincott Williams & Wilkins

CHAPTER 1

Introduction to Pharmacology

■ Exercises

Define the following.

pharmacology _____

_____

_____

biotechnology _____

_____

_____

drug therapy_____

_____

prototypes _____

_____

_____

medications _____

_____

generic drug name _____

_____

_____

systemic drug effects_____

_____

trade drug name _____

_____

_____

synthetic chemical compounds _____

_____

_____

over-the-counter (OTC) _____

_____

_____

Answer in essay form.

1. Explain the advantages of synthetic drugs in relation to pure form drugs.

2. Discuss pharmacoeconomics.

3. Compare the two routes of access to therapeutic drugs.

4. How do you distinguish between trade names and generic names of drugs?

5. How are drugs classified?

Fill in the chart.

Name	Year	Provision
	1970	Regulated distribution of narcotics and other drugs of abuse
Durham-Humphrey		Designated drugs that are prescribed by a physician and dispensed by a pharmacist
Kefauver-Harris Amendment	1962	
	1914	Controlled the manufacture, importation, transportation, and distribution of opium, cocaine, marijuana, and their derivatives
Food, Drug and Cosmetic Act	1938	

Match the following characteristics with the categories of controlled substances.

1. _____ may be dispensed in some states by a pharmacist without a physician's prescription

2. _____ drugs that are not approved for medical use

3. _____ drugs that are used medically and have high abuse potential

4. _____ prescription appetite suppressants except amphetamines

5. _____ abuse of drugs may lead to psychological or physical dependence

6. _____ codeine, morphine, and cocaine

7. _____ heroin, LSD, and marijuana

8. _____ commonly used sedatives and hypnotics

9. _____ drugs that contain moderate amounts of controlled substances

10. _____ drugs with some potential for abuse

a. Schedule I
b. Schedule II
c. Schedule III
d. Schedule IV
e. Schedule V

■ Review Questions

1. Which of the following deals with how drugs are used in the prevention, diagnosis, and treatment of disease?
   a. pharmacokinetics
   b. pharmacotherapy
   c. pharmacogenetics
   d. pharmacodynamics

2. Which law established official standards and requirements for accurate labeling of drugs?
   a. Pure Food and Drug Act of 1906
   b. Food, Drug and Cosmetic Act of 1938
   c. Kefauver-Harris Amendment of 1962
   d. Sherley Amendment

3. The physician has ordered phentermine, an appetite suppressant, for your client. In explaining the potential for abuse, you are aware that this drug is categorized as a:
   a. Schedule II drug
   b. Schedule III drug
   c. Schedule IV drug
   d. Schedule V drug

4. The Food and Drug Administration is responsible for:
   a. obtaining healthy volunteers for initial drug testing
   b. testing new drugs for safety and effectiveness
   c. reviewing drug research studies
   d. marketing new drugs to consumers

5. Most drugs are prescribed for:
   a. local effects
   b. systemic effects
   c. immediate effects
   d. long-term effects

6. Penicillin is the standard by which other antibacterial drugs are compared and is considered a/an:
   a. regulatory drug
   b. experimental drug
   c. prototype drug
   d. placebo-controlled drug

7. Testing of new drugs usually will continue if:
   a. there are excessive side and toxic effects
   b. there is evidence of safety and therapeutic potential
   c. human subjects will participate in a clinical trial
   d. there is an increased number of people who need the drug

8. Which of the following is an advantage of using OTC drugs?
   a. self-diagnosis of an illness
   b. delay in having to seek treatment from health care provider
   c. faster and easier access to effective treatment
   d. insurance coverage for OTC drugs

9. A nurse would know that Schedule II controlled drugs:
   a. must be reordered after 6 months or five refills
   b. may be sold over the counter
   c. may be refilled once with a new prescription
   d. cannot be refilled

10. In studying pharmacology, the most important strategy is to:
    a. focus on therapeutic classifications and their prototypes
    b. memorize all drugs and their side effects
    c. not worry about the therapeutic effects
    d. use only the *Physicians' Desk Reference* as a source for drug information

CHAPTER 2

Basic Concepts and Processes

■ Exercises

Match the following terms with their definitions.

1. ____ pharmacokinetics

2. ____ absorption

3. ____ bioavailability

4. ____ distribution

5. ____ metabolism

6. ____ excretion

7. ____ serum half-life

8. ____ pharmacodynamics

9. ____ receptors

10. ____ agonists

11. ____ antagonists

12. ____ synergism

13. ____ teratogenicity

14. ____ drug tolerance

15. ____ idiosyncracy

a. Drugs that inhibit cell function

b. Unexpected reaction to a drug that occurs the first time it is given

c. Involves drug movement through the body to sites of action

d. The portion of a dose that reaches the systemic circulation and is available to act on body cells

e. The method by which drugs are inactivated or detoxified by the body

f. Refers to elimination of a drug from the body

g. Drugs that produce effects similar to those produced by naturally occurring substances

h. When two drugs with different sites or mechanisms of action produce greater effects when taken together than does either dose when taken alone

i. The process that occurs between the time a drug enters the body and the time it enters the bloodstream to be circulated

j. Occurs when the body becomes accustomed to a drug over time so that a larger dose is required to produce the same effect

k. Involves the transport of drug molecules within the body

l. The time required for the blood concentration of a drug to decrease by 50%

m. Involves drug actions on target cells

n. The ability of a substance to cause abnormal fetal development when taken by pregnant women

o. Proteins located within cells

Place a T (true) or F (false) in each blank.

1. _____ Few drug actions occur at the cellular level.

2. _____ Drugs must reach and interact with the cell membrane in order to produce a cellular function.

3. _____ An intravenous drug is 50% bioavailable.

4. _____ Only the free or unbound portion of a drug acts on body cells.

5. _____ Most drugs are water-soluble.

6. _____ A function of drug metabolism is to convert fat-soluble drugs into water-soluble metabolites.

7. _____ "First-pass effect" is the process that occurs when oral drugs are absorbed from the GI tract and carried to the liver through the portal circulation.

8. _____ Drug action begins when drug levels fall below the minimum effective concentration.

9. _____ A drug with a short half-life requires more frequent administration than one with a long half-life.

10. _____ A large number of receptors must be occupied by drug molecules to produce pharmacologic effects.

11. _____ Pregnancy Category C indicates animal reproduction studies have revealed an adverse effect on the fetus and there are no well-controlled studies in humans.

12. _____ If most receptor sites are occupied, increasing the drug dosage will increase the pharmacologic effect.

13. _____ Impaired kidney and liver function greatly increase the risks of adverse drug effects.

14. _____ The most common mechanism of drug fever is an allergic reaction.

15. _____ Systemic absorption can occur from the mucosa of the rectum.

Define the following.

passive diffusion _____

_____

_____

facilitated diffusion _____

_____

_____

active transport _____

_____

_____

Fill in the chart.

Drug	Antidote
heparin	
	naloxone (Narcan)
	diphenhydramine HCL (Benadryl)
warfarin (Coumadin)	
	acetylcysteine (Mucomyst)
beta blockers	

■ Review Questions

1. When caring for the elderly, the nurse is aware that the effect of aging on the liver results in:
   a. reduced intensity of drug effects
   b. reduced incidence of toxicity
   c. prolonged drug effects
   d. inadequate blood levels of a drug

2. Vistaril, given in combination with Talwin, counteracts the side effects of nausea caused by the Talwin. The drug–drug interaction responsible for the desired effect is:
   a. addition
   b. antagonism
   c. synergism
   d. potentiation

3. On the 2 AM round, the nurse finds a client restless and unable to sleep. A sedative-hypnotic is administered. Two hours later, the nurse finds the client irritable and restless. This is characteristic of:
   a. an allergic reaction
   b. a teratogenic effect
   c. a tachyphalactic reaction
   d. an idiosyncratic response

4. A client is receiving an antibiotic for an infection. The nurse teaches the client that taking most drugs with food will:
   a. have no effect on the physiological action of the drug
   b. increase the rate of absorption of the drug
   c. decrease the amount of drug being absorbed
   d. increase appetite

5. Your client has a drug level of 100 units/mL. The drug's half-life is 2 hours. If concentrations above 50 units/mL are toxic and no further drug is given, how long will it take for the blood level to reach the nontoxic range?
   a. 1 hour
   b. 2 hours
   c. 4 hours
   d. 5 hours

6. Thyroid disorders mostly affect which pharmacokinetic function?
   a. absorption
   b. distribution
   c. metabolism
   d. excretion

7. Which of the following clients will a nurse expect to experience alterations in drug metabolism?
   a. a 52-year-old male with cirrhosis of the liver
   b. a 35-year-old female with ulcerative colitis
   c. a 41-year-old male with cancer of the stomach
   d. a 60-year-old female with acute renal failure

8. Your client has been taking a medication for several months for chronic back pain. He tells you that the medication is no longer relieving the pain. In discussing this with the client, you explain the possibility of:
   a. drug fever
   b. diffusion
   c. drug tolerance
   d. hypersensitivity

9. The process of the movement of a drug from the place it enters the body until it reaches the circulation is which of the following pharmacokinetic activities?
   a. absorption
   b. distribution
   c. metabolism
   d. excretion

10. The amount of a drug that gets into the circulation and is available to the tissues is referred to as:
    a. bioavailability
    b. cumulative toxicity
    c. serum half-life
    d. detoxification

CHAPTER 3

Dosage Calculations

■ Exercises

Fill in the blank.

1. Almost all medication orders are written using the _____ system.

2. _____ express biologic activity in animal tests for drug dosage.

3. _____ express ionic activity of a drug.

4. The metric system is a _____ system.

5. The _____ system may be used by clients at home.

6. _____ _____ is used for pediatric dosages and is based on weight.

7. A more accurate method of dosage calculation for children is based on _____ _____ ____.

8. The _____ _____ is the number of drops per milliliter that an intravenous administration set delivers.

9. The drop factor for all micro drip administration sets is ____ drops per mL.

10. The _____ and _____ systems may be used for liquid dosage administration.

Fill in the blank with the approximate equivalent.

1. 1 kg = _____ lb

2. 1 g = _____mg

3. 60 mg = _____gr

4. 1 mL = _____ cc

5. 1 cc = _____ minims

6. 1 cup = _____ mL

7. 1 mg = _____mcg

8. 30 mg = _____oz

9. 1 dram = _____mL

10. 15 gtt = _____ mL

Convert each item to the equivalent.

1. 30 drops = ____minims

2. 50 lbs = ____kg

3. 2 drams = ____mL

4. 3500 mg = ____g

5. 2.5 tsp = ____mL

6. 12 mL = ____cc

7. 2 L = ____mL

8. 32 minims = ____cc

9. 500 mL = ____cups

10. 2.5 mg = ____mcg

Calculate the following drug dosages.

1. Order: Tegretol 800 mg/d
   Label: Tegretol XL 200 mg/tablet
   How many tablets will the client take each day?

2. Order: Benadryl elixir 25 mg
   Label: Benadryl elixir 12.5 mg per 5 mL
   How much medication will you administer?

3. Order: KCL 40 mEq PO
   Label: KCL 10 mEq/15 mL
   How many mL will you administer?

4. Order: Heparin 1500 units IV
   Label: Heparin 1000 units/mL
   How much heparin will you administer?

5. Order: Synthroid 50 mcg PO daily
   Label: Synthroid 0.025 mg/tablet
   How many tablets will you administer?

6. Robitussin cough syrup 600 mg in 1 oz is available. The order is for 225 mg. How many cc should you administer?

7. Keflex is available in 250-mg capsules. Keflex 0.5 gm PO is ordered. How many capsules should you administer?

8. Prepare penicillin 600,000 units IM. Penicillin 1,200,000 units/mL is available. How many mL will you administer?

9. Demerol 50 mg/mL is available. The order is for Demerol 100 mg. How many mL will you administer?

10. Maalox 1/2 oz is ordered. How many cc would you administer?

CHAPTER 4

Administering Medications

■ Exercises

Answer the following.

1. Define the "seven rights."

2. Explain why the nurse is legally responsible for safe and accurate administration of medication.

3. List all the components of a medication order.

4. Define the term *parenteral*.

5. Explain why controlled-release tablets and capsules should never be broken or crushed.

Place a T (true) or F (false) in each blank.

1. _____ A nurse should never question a physician if a drug order is unclear.

2. _____ When calculating a child's drug dosage, always ask a pharmacist or another nurse to do the calculation also and compare the results.

3. _____ Needleless systems reduce the spread of blood-borne pathogens.

4. _____ A nurse is not legally responsible for actions delegated to other health care personnel.

5. _____ Only the nurse is responsible for getting medication to a client.

6. _____ Unit dose wrappings of oral drugs should be left with the medication until the nurse is in the presence of the client and is ready to administer the drug.

7. _____ Nurses may take verbal or telephone orders from physicians.

8. _____ Some drugs are available in one dosage form only.

9. _____ Enteric-coated tablets delay absorption until the medication reaches the stomach.

10. _____ Single-dose vials contain preservatives and should be kept for other dosages after initial use.

11. _____ The term *gauge* refers to the lumen size of the needle.

12. _____ A 22-gauge 1½ inch needle is used for subcutaneous injections.

Match the abbreviations with the appropriate terms.

1. ____ cubic centimeter
2. ____ before meals
3. ____ right eye
4. ____ by mouth
5. ____ drops
6. ____ immediately
7. ____ when needed
8. ____ after meals
9. ____ daily
10. ____ every 4 hours
11. ____ left eye
12. ____ bedtime
13. ____ twice daily
14. ____ as desired
15. ____ four times daily

a. OS
b. PRN
c. pc
d. qd
e. PO
f. q 4h
g. cc
h. ad lib
i. stat
j. OD
k. hs
l. bid
m. ac
n. qid
o. gtt

■ Review Questions

1. The client is to receive ampicillin 500 mg PO tid ac. Which of the following reflects proper scheduling?
   a. 4 AM, 12 noon, 8 PM
   b. 7 AM, 11 AM, 6 PM
   c. 7 AM, 1 PM, 8 PM
   d. 8 AM, 12 noon, 4 PM, 8 PM

2. A client asks the nurse whether he can divide his enteric-coated tablet in half. The nurse tells him not to because dividing the drug will:
   a. make the drug less potent
   b. cause severe abdominal cramps
   c. alter the drug's absorption
   d. produce no therapeutic effect

3. The client is a 4-year-old who has a temperature of 103° and is vomiting. The physician has ordered Tylenol for the fever. The nurse would administer the Tylenol in which of the following forms?
   a. liquid
   b. lozenge
   c. tablet
   d. suppository

4. The nurse is assigned to administer medication to 10 clients. Which of the following would be the initial action of the nurse before preparing the medications?
   a. Identify the client by asking him what his name is.
   b. Wash his hands.
   c. Explain the action of the medications to the client.
   d. Record the administration of the medication.

5. Which of the following statements best describes the reason for aspiration before injecting medication into a muscle?
   a. to determine whether the needle is in the correct muscle
   b. to decrease discomfort
   c. to avoid major nerves in the area
   d. to avoid injecting the medication into a blood vessel

6. The client is 15 months old and is hospitalized for pneumonia. The nurse will administer an intramuscular injection in which of the following muscles?
   a. deltoid
   b. dorsogluteal muscle
   c. ventrogluteal muscle
   d. vastus lateralis

7. The term for IV administration of a drug over 15 to 60 minutes is called:
   a. a loading dose
   b. an IVP (push)
   c. a peripheral IV infusion
   d. an IVPB (piggyback)

8. Which of the following is proper placement of the needle for an intramuscular injection into the dorsogluteal site?

    a. below the greater trochanter and posterior iliac spine

    b. above and inside a diagonal line drawn from the greater trochanter of the femur to the anterior superior iliac crest

    c. below the anterior superior iliac spine and above the greater trochanter

    d. above and outside a diagonal line drawn from the greater trochanter of the femur to the posterior superior iliac spine

9. Which of the following is true regarding administration of medications by the oral route?

    a. It is convenient and relatively inexpensive.

    b. Oral administration is best for all clients.

    c. Gastrointestinal upset rarely occurs.

    d. Water given with medication retards drug absorption.

10. The nurse is to administer gentamicin gtt 2 OD. The nurse will administer the drug in the client's:

    a. right eye

    b. left eye

    c. right ear

    d. left ear

CHAPTER 5

Nursing Process in Drug Therapy

■ Exercises

Fill in the blank.

1. The _____ _____ is a systematic method used to gather data to plan and implement client care and evaluate the outcomes of that care.

2. Nurses plan and provide client care based on _____ data.

3. Client goals should be stated in terms of _____ behavior.

4. _____ can be evaluated soon after drug administration or after longer periods of time.

5. Nursing responsibility related to drug therapy may be designated in _____ _____ _____.

Answer the following.

1. Give an example of a nursing diagnosis related to drug therapy.

2. List three examples of expected outcomes related to prescribed drug therapy.

3. List five areas of nursing intervention in relation to drug therapy.

4. List five examples of interventions that decrease the need for drug therapy.

5. Explain why client teaching related to drug therapy is important.

6. Why do nurses have difficulties in evaluating outcomes of drug therapy?

7. List five questions a nurse should ask when assessing a client's medication history.

8. Discuss current legislation in regard to herbal and dietary supplements.

9. What are the two major concerns that health care providers have concerning the use of herbal and dietary supplements?

10. What must be considered in pediatric drug therapy?

Place a T (true) or F (false) in each blank.

1. ____ The goal of drug therapy should be to minimize beneficial effects and maximize adverse effects.

2. ____ Drugs should not be prescribed for conditions for which nondrug measures are effective.

3. ____ Few variables influence a drug's effect on the body.

4. ____ Decreasing the number of drugs and the frequency of administration increases the client's compliance with prescribed drugs.

5. ____ Fixed-dose drug combinations are commonly used.

6. ____ The smallest amount of the most potent drug for therapeutic benefit should be given.

7. ____ Clients with severe kidney disease often need smaller doses of drugs that are excreted by the kidneys.

8. ____ A physician may order a loading dose of a drug if it has a short half-life.

9. ____ Drug therapy is less predictable in children than in adults.

10. ____ Older adults are usually less likely to metabolize and excrete drugs efficiently.

11. ____ For elderly clients receiving long-term drug therapy at home, childproof containers should be avoided.

12. ____ Liver impairment does not interfere with drug metabolism.

13. ____ Alcohol is toxic to the liver and increases the risk of hepatotoxicity.

14. ____ Serum creatinine is a reliable indicator of renal function when determining drug dosage.

15. ____ For a critically ill client, therapeutic drug effects may be increased.

Match uses to herbal and dietary supplements. Some uses may be used more than once.

1. ____ chamomile

2. ____ feverfew

3. ____ ginkgo biloba

4. ____ garlic

5. ____ echinacea

6. ____ ginseng

7. ____ glucosamine

8. ____ black cohosh

9. ____ chondroitin

10. ____ ephedra

11. ____ Saint John's wort

12. ____ saw palmetto

13. ____ melatonin

14. ____ valerian

15. ____ kava

a. Weight loss

b. Arthritis

c. Insomnia

d. Depression

e. Abdominal cramping

f. High cholesterol

g. Menopausal symptoms

h. Stamina and strength

i. Urinary symptoms

j. Common cold

k. Anxiety and stress

l. Memory

m. Migraines

■ Clinical Challenge

Your 88-year-old client is being discharged from the hospital with a newly prescribed drug. Formulate a topical outline for a teaching plan you would use in this clinical situation.

■ Review Questions

1. A client is being discharged on an antibiotic and has very little knowledge concerning the drug. Which of the following best reflects an expected goal of client-teaching related to the antibiotic?

   a. Client will be able to interpret culture and sensitivity test.

   b. Family members will understand the physiological action of the antibiotic.

   c. Client will exercise three times a week.

   d. Client will be able to identify two adverse effects of the antibiotic.

2. A 62-year-old client has just been diagnosed as having diabetes mellitus. Before giving him any medication, the nurse must first assess all of the following except:

   a. medications taken at home

   b. other medical conditions that may interfere with drug therapy for the diabetes mellitus

   c. medication allergies

   d. his response to the new medication

3. A client is in the cardiac care unit following a mild cardiac infarction. She is on multiple drug therapy, including three intramuscular (IM) injections per day. Which of the following would be the appropriate nursing diagnosis related to the administration of the IM injections?

   a. altered nutrition: more than body requirements related to overeating

   b. anxiety related to three IM injections each day

   c. impaired social interaction related to being in the cardiac care unit

   d. noncompliance related to overuse of medication

4. Which statement by the client with heart disease would indicate that health teaching related to medication was ineffective?

   a. "It's best to take my medication as the doctor ordered."

   b. "It shouldn't matter that I skip a couple of doses now and then."

   c. "I will call the clinic if I experience any side effects from my medications."

   d. "I will get all of my medications at the same pharmacy."

5. During drug therapy, clients with liver disease are monitored for which of the following?

   a. dizziness

   b. jaundice

   c. headache

   d. constipation

6. The goal of drug therapy in critically ill clients is to:

   a. support vital functions to relieve life-threatening symptoms

   b. decrease medication use to minimize client cost

   c. disregard laboratory tests related to the client's physiological condition

   d. increase or decrease dietary intake, depending on weight of the client

7. Which of the following herbal/dietary supplements could increase the potential for bleeding when taking aspirin?

   a. melatonin

   b. saw palmetto

   c. ginseng

   d. chondroitin

8. When implementing medication therapy for a client, the nurse is responsible for which of the following actions?

   a. changing the drug dosage if side effects occur

   b. discontinuing the drug if the client does not want to take it

   c. sharing information concerning therapeutic value of the drug in other clients

   d. checking for the correct dosage of the drug prior to administration

9. Which phase of the nursing process requires the nurse to formulate a client outcome related to the administration of medication?

   a. assessment

   b. planning

   c. implementation

   d. evaluation

10. In gathering assessment data from a medication history, which of the following would be most helpful to the nurse in planning client care?

    a. the name of the pharmacist the client talks to regarding his medication

    b. a list of all prescribed and over-the-counter medications and herbal and dietary supplements the client takes

    c. the medication history of the client's mother

    d. dietary intake for 1 day

CHAPTER 6

Narcotic Analgesics and Narcotic Antagonists

■ Exercises

Match the following.

1. _____ thalamus

2. _____ patient-controlled analgesia

3. _____ methadone (Dolophine)

4. _____ oxycodone (Roxicodone)

5. _____ opioid peptides

6. _____ fentanyl (Duragesic)

7. _____ bradykinin

8. _____ tramadol (Ultram)

9. _____ butorphanol (Stadol)

10. _____ pentazocine (Talwin)

a. Pain-producing substance
b. A popular drug of abuse, which has lead to deaths and criminal activity
c. A transdermal formulation used to treat chronic pain
d. Relay station for incoming stimuli
e. Used to treat fibromyalgia
f. Not recommended in children younger than 18 years of age
g. Interact with opiate receptors to inhibit pain transmission
h. Used in the detoxification and maintenance treatment of opiate addicts
i. Adverse effects include hallucinations and bizarre dreams
j. Allows for self-administration of medication

Answer the following.

1. Describe the process that must occur for a person to feel pain.

2. Define endogenous analgesia system.

3. Explain the physiological action of a narcotic analgesic.

4. List pharmacological effects of narcotic analgesics.

5. Why would narcotic analgesics be contraindicated in a client with chronic lung disease?

6. Explain how narcotic agonists/antagonists work in the body.

7. Describe the physiological action of narcotic antagonists.

8. Explain the concept of morphine as a "nonceiling" drug.

9. Why does a dose of an oral narcotic analgesic need to be larger than an injected dose?

10. List characteristics of narcotic withdrawal.

Place a T (true) or F (false) in each blank.

1. ____ In chronic pain, narcotic analgesics are most effective when given parenterally.

2. ____ Morphine (sulfate), given in combination with cimetidine (Tagamet), may increase CNS and respiratory depression.

3. ____ A narcotic analgesic, given in combination with an antihypertensive drug, may cause hypertension.

4. ____ Clients taking naltrexone (ReVia) do not respond to narcotic analgesics if pain control is needed.

5. ____ The drug of choice in treatment of narcotic overdose is naloxone (Narcan).

6. ____ Codeine produces stronger analgesic and antitussive effects than morphine.

7. ____ An injection of 200 mg of meperidine (Demerol) is equivalent to 10 mg of morphine.

8. ____ Referred pain is pain occurring from tissue damage in one area of the body but felt in another area.

9. ____ Morphine is often the drug of choice for severe pain.

10. ____ Narcotic analgesics are commonly used to manage pain associated with disease processes and invasive diagnostic and therapeutic procedures.

■Clinical Challenge

Discuss the difference in pain management in a client in acute pain who is 1 day post-operative from hip replacement surgery and a client who is experiencing chronic cancer pain.

■Review Questions

1. It may be necessary to repeat doses of naloxone (Narcan) to a client who has had too much morphine because the narcotic antagonist:
   a. has less strength in each dose than do individual doses of morphine
   b. has a shorter half-life than does morphine
   c. combined with morphine, increases the physiological action of the morphine
   d. causes the respiratory rate to decrease

2. Which of the following would indicate a therapeutic effect of a narcotic analgesic for a client who has been experiencing severe pain?

   a. restlessness during the night hours

   b. increased participation in AM care activities

   c. shorter intervals between medication administration

   d. increased facial grimacing during movement

3. Before administering a narcotic analgesic, the initial action of the nurse would be to:

   a. check the apical pulse and compare it with the radial pulse

   b. check the blood pressure lying and standing

   c. check the temperature

   d. check the rate, depth, and rhythm of respirations

4. Codeine given with acetaminophen produces which of the following effects:

   a. additive

   b. synergistic

   c. cumulative

   d. antagonistic

5. Your post-op client will be receiving hydromorphone (Dilaudid) via patient-controlled analgesia (PCA) and is having second thoughts about administering his own medication for fear of overdosing himself. A nursing diagnosis for your client would be:

   a. knowledge deficient related to the use of PCA

   b. impaired gas exchange related to the surgery

   c. anxiety related to surgical procedure

   d. impaired judgment related to increased dosage of medication

6. Your client is to receive propoxyphene (Darvon) as needed for pain. Which of the following would be an appropriate medication order for your client?

   a. 390 mg qid IM

   b. 65 mg q 4h PRN PO

   c. 65 mg bid PRN PO

   d. 100 mg q 2h PO

7. You have just administered an IM injection of meperidine (Demerol) to your client. The most important nursing measure you should perform before leaving the room should be to:

   a. close the draperies

   b. make sure the side rails are up

   c. ask all the visitors to leave the room

   d. offer your client something to drink

8. A common side effect of a narcotic analgesic is:

   a. constipation

   b. diarrhea

   c. increased respirations

   d. fine hand tremors

9. You suspect that the neonate you will be receiving in the newborn intensive care unit may be experiencing narcotic withdrawal. You will most likely see signs and symptoms that include:

   a. tremors

   b. decreased muscle tone

   c. lethargy

   d. bradycardia

10. An automatic "stop order" for narcotics is usually between:

    a. 24 and 36 hours

    b. 48 and 72 hours

    c. 60 and 96 hours

    d. 72 and 130 hours

CHAPTER 7

Analgesic–Antipyretic–Anti-inflammatory and Related Drugs

■ Exercises

Match the following terms with their definitions.

1. ____ pyrogens
2. ____ chondroitin
3. ____ tinnitus
4. ____ prostaglandins
5. ____ histamine
6. ____ glucosamine
7. ____ bradykinin
8. ____ Reye's syndrome
9. ____ inflammation
10. ____ cyclooxygenases

a. Normal body response to tissue damage
b. Enzymes required for prostaglandin formation
c. Normal component of joint cartilage
d. Chemical mediators found in most body tissue
e. Ringing or roaring in the ears
f. First chemical mediator released in the inflammatory response
g. Essential structural component of joint connective tissue
h. A kinin in body fluids that becomes physiologically active with tissue injury
i. Fever-producing agent
j. A disease seen in children under 15 associated with use of aspirin

Place a T (true) or F (false) in each blank.

1. ____ The first drug of choice for a moderate to severe migraine attack is ergotamine tartrate/caffeine (Cafergot).

2. ____ When allopurinol (Zyloprim) is taken for gout, uric acid blood levels decrease to normal range within 1 to 3 weeks.

3. ____ You must take acetaminophen with food.

4. ____ If one nonsteroidal anti-inflammatory drug (NSAID) is not effective, another one may produce therapeutic effects.

5. ____ Over-the-counter (OTC) ibuprofen is the same medication as prescription Motrin.

6. ____ Anticoagulants decrease the effects of indomethacin (Indocin).

7. ____ Symptoms of ergot poisoning include coolness, numbness and tingling of extremities, vomiting, and dizziness.

8. ____ Celecoxib (Celebrex) should be taken with food.

9. ____ Aspirin toxicity occurs at levels above 500 mcg/mL.

10. ____ In older adults, long-term use of NSAIDs can increase the risk of serious gastrointestinal bleeding.

Match the trade names with the following generic drugs.

1. ____ celecoxib
2. ____ etodolac
3. ____ nabumetone
4. ____ naproxen sodium
5. ____ sulindac
6. ____ sumatriptan
7. ____ acetaminophen

8. ____ allopurinol

9. ____ ibuprofen

10. ____ rofecoxib

a. Motrin

b. Vioxx

c. Tylenol

d. Zyloprim

e. Lodine

f. Anaprox

g. Imitrex

h. Celebrex

i. Clinoril

j. Relafen

■ Clinical Challenge

Your client is brought into the emergency department complaining of nausea, vomiting, fever, tinnitus, and blurred vision. During your initial assessment, you determine that the client is mildly confused. You are aware that he has rheumatoid arthritis. What do you think his medical diagnosis will be? What would be your plan of care?

■ Review Questions

1. Your client is 9 years old and has symptoms of influenza. Her mother explains that her fever has been between 102° and 103° for the last 2 days. Which medication would you suggest be given to her?

   a. acetaminophen

   b. aspirin

   c. naproxen

   d. nabumetone

2. Your client has been diagnosed with rheumatoid arthritis. He has been placed on celecoxib (Celebrex) 100 mg tid. You will provide your client with the following information about this drug:

   a. Expect heart palpitations to occur.

   b. Take with food to decrease gastric irritation.

   c. Increase the dosage if prescribed dosage does not provide relief.

   d. Wear sunscreen when outside, due to hypersensitivity effect.

3. The emergency department nurse is expecting a client to be brought in who is exhibiting signs and symptoms of acetaminophen poisoning. The nurse will have the following drug available for administration when the client arrives:

   a. oxaprozin (Daypro)

   b. vitamin K

   c. acetylcysteine (Mucomyst)

   d. naloxone (Narcan)

4. Your client has been on naproxen (Naprosyn) for some time. When evaluating him on his return visits to the clinic, you will monitor which of the following?

   a. low-density lipoprotein

   b. serum amylase level

   c. blood glucose level

   d. bleeding time

5. Your client is to begin colchicine therapy for acute gout. You inform him that, with oral therapy, he should have pain relief within:

   a. 2 to 4 hours

   b. 6 to 12 hours

   c. 12 to 20 hours

   d. 24 to 48 hours

6. Your client has a history of migraines. She has just been given a prescription for sumatriptan (Imitrex). Which symptoms would you tell her to report to her physician immediately?

   a. decreased appetite

   b. chest pain

   c. slight weight gain

   d. fatigue

7. Which of the following statements by your client reveals a potential problem with NSAID therapy?

    a. "I take my medication with a full glass of water."

    b. "I can still have my glass of wine every night."

    c. "I should make sure my doctor checks for blood in my stool."

    d. "I have problems with swallowing, but I do not crush my tablets."

8. Your client is on an antigout drug. Your teaching plan concerning this drug in preventing the formation of uric acid kidney stones would involve which of the following?

    a. Walk at least 2 miles three times a week.

    b. Take on an empty stomach.

    c. Avoid exposure to sunlight.

    d. Drink 2 to 3 quarts of water daily.

9. A 72-year-old man has been taking a baby aspirin every day for the last 5 years. He is scheduled for major dental work in 1 month. It will be important for this man to:

    a. double the amount of aspirin he is taking

    b. avoid aspirin for 2 weeks prior to the dental procedure

    c. increase his fluid intake by 1000 cc per day 1 week prior to the dental work

    d. expect complications following the dental work

10. Your 65-year-old client has been diagnosed with osteoarthritis of the hands and feet. She reveals to you that she is having difficulty performing light housework. Which of the following would be an appropriate nursing diagnosis related to her complaint?

    a. risk for injury related to adverse drug effects

    b. activity intolerance related to pain

    c. knowledge deficient related to medical diagnosis

    d. altered nutrition related to medication

CHAPTER 8

Antianxiety and Sedative-Hypnotic Drugs

■ Exercises

Match the following terms with their definitions.

1. ____ sedative

2. ____ alprazolam (Xanax)

3. ____ kava

4. ____ midazolam (Versed)

5. ____ hypnotic

6. ____ sertraline (Zoloft)

7. ____ flumazenil

8. ____ zaleplon (Sonata)

9. ____ diazepam (Valium)

10. ____ chlordiazepoxide (Librium)

a. Herbal/dietary supplement that suppresses emotional excitability

b. Antidote for benzodiazepines

c. Prototype benzodiazepine

d. Produces sleep

e. Prescribed for obsessive-compulsive disorder

f. An oral nonbenzodiazepine that should be used with caution in Japanese clients

g. Prescribed in acute alcohol withdrawal

h. Promotes relaxation

i. Preoperative sedation used for short-term treatment of anxiety

j. Benzodiazepine used for panic disorder

Answer the following.

1. Why is buspirone preferred over a benzodiazepine?

2. Explain the pharmacokinetics of benzodiazepines.

3. List contraindications to benzodiazepines.

4. Compare buspirone and benzodiazepines.

5. What is the goal for treatment for insomnia?

Place the generic name in the blank next to the trade name.

1. Librium _____

2. Ambien _____

3. Versed _____

4. BuSpar _____

5. Vistaril _____

6. Xanax _____

7. Sonata _____

8. Zoloft _____

9. Ativan _____

10. Restoril _____

Place T (true) or F (false) in each blank.

1. ____ Midazolam (Versed) may be mixed in the same syringe with morphine sulfate.

2. ____ At bedtime, food should be taken with zolpidem (Ambien).

3. ____ Cimetidine (Tagamet) decreases the effects of zaleplon (Sonata).

4. ____ Narcotic analgesics increase effects of antianxiety and sedative-hypnotic drugs.

5. ____ Diazepam (Valium) is physically incompatible with other drugs.

6. ____ Benzodiazepines can be given intramuscularly in the deltoid muscle.

7. ____ Adverse effects of antianxiety and sedative-hypnotic drugs are caused by central nervous system depression.

8. ____ Excessive drowsiness is more likely to occur when drug therapy begins.

9. ____ Lorazepam (Ativan) is probably the benzodiazepine of first choice.

10. ____ To prevent withdrawal symptoms, benzodiazepines should be tapered in dose and gradually discontinued.

■ Clinical Challenge

Your client has been taking a benzodiazepine for 4 months. During his most recent clinic visit, you suspect that he has stopped taking the drug. What symptoms would you assess for? What would you tell him regarding discontinuing the drug?

■ Review Questions

1. Your client describes having feelings of fear and impending doom. She states that she has palpitations, shortness of breath, and sometimes dizziness and nausea. Your assessment indicates that she is having panic attacks. The most appropriate drug for your client is:

   a. hydroxyzine (Vistaril)

   b. buspirone (BuSpar)

   c. alprazolam (Xanax)

   d. lorazepam (Ativan)

2. Which of the following statements by your client indicates his understanding of his new drug, buspirone (BuSpar)?

   a. "My muscles are so relaxed after I take my medication."

   b. "BuSpar will cause me to go to sleep after I take each dose."

   c. "BuSpar gave me immediate relief the first day I took it."

   d. "It will probably take 3 to 4 weeks for my new medication to make me feel better."

3. Which of the following nondrug measures would you implement to enhance the effectiveness of an antianxiety drug?

   a. Turn out bright lights and decrease the temperature.

   b. Do not worry your client with details concerning his care.

   c. Spend at least 30 minutes explaining how his antianxiety drug will decrease his anxiety.

   d. Withhold all other medications.

4. Your client is drowsy, and his speech is slurred. He appears to have difficulty concentrating. You suspect that he is experiencing:

   a. a panic attack

   b. sleep deprivation

   c. obsessive-compulsive disorder

   d. hyperactivity

5. Which of the following drugs will decrease the effects of an antianxiety agent?

   a. nicotine

   b. alcohol

   c. cimetidine

   d. oral contraceptives

6. Your client is to receive a hypnotic for the first time. You will tell her to expect drowsiness within:

    a. 10 minutes

    b. 15 minutes

    c. 30 minutes

    d. 60 minutes

7. Which of the following is not a side effect of an antianxiety medication?

    a. hypertension

    b. hypotension

    c. confusion

    d. impaired mobility

8. When administering a sedative, you encourage your client to drink a full glass of water. When he questions you about the amount of water, the most appropriate response would be:

    a. "The water is necessary to dilute the drug."

    b. "The water increases dissolution and absorption of the drug for a faster onset of action."

    c. "The more fluid you drink, the faster the elimination of the drug from the body."

    d. "The fluid helps decrease the irritation to the body tissues."

9. If a client is excessively sedated at the time of the next sedative dose, you should:

    a. omit the dose and record the reason

    b. withhold the dose for 30 minutes

    c. administer flumazenil

    d. have the physician discontinue the drug

10. Your client has cirrhosis. Which of the following antianxiety agents would be appropriate for her?

    a. temazepam (Restoril)

    b. lorazepam (Ativan)

    c. buspirone (BuSpar)

    d. zaleplon (Sonata)

CHAPTER 9

Antipsychotic Drugs

■ Exercises

Place T (true) or F (false) in each blank.

1. ____ Increased salivation is a common side effect of antipsychotic drugs.

2. ____ Antacids should not be taken with antipsychotic drugs.

3. ____ Most adverse effects are less likely to occur or be severe with the newer "atypical" drugs than with phenothiazines.

4. ____ Delusions indicate severe mental illness.

5. ____ Overt psychotic symptoms must be present for at least 12 months before a diagnosis of schizophrenia can be made.

6. ____ Symptoms of schizophrenia may begin gradually or suddenly.

7. ____ Overactivity of dopamine accounts for negative symptoms of schizophrenia.

8. ____ Chlorpromazine (Thorazine) was the first drug to treat psychotic disorders effectively.

9. ____ Phenothiazines may cause psychological dependence but do not cause physical dependence.

10. ____ "Atypical" antipsychotic drugs have become the first drug of choice.

Answer the following.

1. List positive symptoms of schizophrenia.

2. List negative symptoms of schizophrenia.

3. Describe the difference between "typical" antipsychotics and "atypical" antipsychotics.

4. List clinical indications for phenothiazines, other than psychiatric illnesses.

5. Why is clozapine (Clozaril) considered a second-line drug?

Fill in the blank.

1. _____ may cause life-threatening agranulocytosis.

2. Antipsychotic drugs bind to dopamine receptors and block the action of _____.

3. The major clinical indication for use of antipsychotic drugs is_____.

4. _____ may be used as the initial drug for treating psychotic disorders.

5. _____ is approved only for the treatment of Tourette's syndrome.

6. The prototype of "atypical" agents is _____.

7. _____ is an antipsychotic drug that is used only for its antiemetic, sedative, and antihistaminic effects.

8. _____ is indicated only when other antipsychotic drugs are ineffective because of its association with cardiac dysrhythmias.

9. _____ _____ are more likely to occur with the older antipsychotic drugs than with the newer "atypical" agents.

10. _____ is considered a hypersensitivity reaction associated with phenothiazines.

■ Clinical Challenge

Your client is a 58-year-old male who has a long-term history of schizophrenia. He has had frequent readmissions to the psychiatric unit. What assessment data do you need to obtain? Based on the frequent readmissions to the hospital, what would you discuss with your client?

■ Review Questions

1. Your client is a newly diagnosed schizophrenic. Which of the following drugs will his physician most likely prescribe for him?
   a. pimozide (Orap)
   b. risperidone (Risperdal)
   c. sotalol (Betapace)
   d. thioridazine hydrochloride (Mellaril)

2. Which of the following clients would be more likely to experience tardive dyskinesia?
   a. a 32-year-old African American male who is taking risperidone (Risperdal)
   b. a 24-year-old Asian female who has taken haloperidol (Haldol) for 2 weeks
   c. an 18-year-old Caucasian male who has just started loxapine (Loxitane) therapy
   d. a 50-year-old Hispanic female who has taken ziprasidone (Geodon) for 2 years

3. A 28-year-old male was hospitalized 1 week ago for acute psychotic symptoms. He is taking quetiapine (Seroquel) daily. He will least likely experience:
   a. extrapyramidal reactions
   b. hypotension
   c. weight gain
   d. sedation

4. You are talking to the mother of a 19-year-old boy who is exhibiting hostility and hyperactivity, and is very combative. The physician explained that her son is probably experiencing an acute psychosis and will be started on an antipsychotic drug. She asks you how long his agitated behavior will last. An appropriate response would be:
   a. "It will be several weeks before he calms down."
   b. "He will always appear agitated."
   c. "I'm not sure. It's really hard to tell."
   d. "Your son should become less agitated a few hours after the drug therapy is started."

5. Your client has been taking an antacid for 2 months. Her physician prescribes loxapine (Loxitane) for acute psychosis. You understand that the dosage of Loxitane may more than likely be:
   a. 10 mg tid PO
   b. decreased because she is taking an antacid
   c. 250 mg/day because of the antacid
   d. increased because of the interaction with the antacid

6. Your client is taking a phenothiazine. Which of the following extrapyramidal reactions indicates involuntary, rhythmic body movements?
   a. dyskinesias
   b. tardive dyskinesia
   c. akathisia
   d. parkinsonism

7. Phenothiazines cause all of the following effects in the body except:
   a. central nervous system depression
   b. hypersensitivity reactions
   c. increase in blood pressure
   d. decrease in body temperature

8. Your client is a newly diagnosed schizophrenic and has been started on risperidone (Risperdal). Which of the following could contribute to non-compliance with his drug therapy?
   a. multiple daily doses of risperidone
   b. high cost of his medication
   c. unpleasant odor of the medication
   d. nausea that occurs after each dose of the medication

9. Your client is on chlorpromazine (Thorazine). For the last 2 days, his blood pressure has been 100/70. He has complained of dizziness and weakness, and has not wanted to get out of bed. Which of the following would be an appropriate nursing diagnosis for him?
   a. impaired physical mobility related to sedation
   b. risk of injury related to excessive sedation
   c. altered tissue perfusion related to hypotension
   d. self-care deficit related to psychosis

10. Which of the following side effects would you look for in a client who is taking ziprasidone (Geodon)?
    a. constipation
    b. hypertension
    c. agitation
    d. diarrhea

CHAPTER 10

Drugs for Mood Disorders: Antidepressants and Mood Stabilizers

■ Exercises

Answer the following.

1. Define monoamine neurotransmitter dysfunction associated with depression.

2. Discuss neuroendocrine factors in relation to depression.

3. List three other factors that may contribute to depression.

4. List the three types of antidepressant drugs.

5. Explain the mechanism of action for antidepressant drugs.

6. List foods that contain tyramine, which should be avoided when taking a monoamine oxidase inhibitor (MAOI).

7. List factors considered in antidepressant drug selection.

8. Why are selective serotonin reuptake inhibitors (SSRIs) considered first-choice drugs?

9. Why should clients be given only a 5- to 7-day supply of antidepressants?

10. Describe a tricyclic antidepressant (TCA) overdose.

Fill in the blank.

1. Toxicity occurs with serum lithium levels above _____ mEq/L.

2. _____ is used to help stop smoking.

3. _____ is considered the most common mental illness.

4. Phenothiazines increase the effects of lithium and may increase the risk of _____.

5. _____ and _____ have little effect on blood sugar levels.

6. Antidepressant effects are due to changes in _____, rather than changes in neurotransmitters.

7. _____ are considered third-line drugs.

8. _____ is the prototype of SSRIs.

9. _____ is not metabolized by the body and is entirely excreted by the kidneys.

10. _____ _____ _____ is a self-prescribed herb that is used for depression.

List adverse effects under each antidepressant group.

TCAs	SSRIs	MAOIs

Match the drug trade name to the generic name.

1. ____ citalopram

2. ____ bupropion

3. ____ amitriptyline

4. ____ mirtazapine

5. ____ imipramine

6. ____ trazodone

7. ____ paroxetine

8. ____ sertraline

9. ____ nefazodone

10. ____ fluoxetine

a. Tofranil

b. Remeron

c. Prozac

d. Paxil

e. Elavil

f. Celexa

g. Serzone

h. Desyrel

i. Zoloft

j. Wellbutrin

■ Clinical Challenge

Your client is unable to concentrate as you talk with him concerning his treatment plan. He interrupts you numerous times as you try to talk with him about his new medication. He is constantly getting up from his chair and walking around the room. He jumps from one topic to another as you continue to talk with him. He tells you that he knows as much as the doctor does about his problems and that you are taking care of the next president of the United States. From your observations, you suspect that your client has which type of mood disorder? He will more than likely be placed on which drug? How long will it take for his medication to decrease his exhibiting behavior?

▪ Review Questions

1. Your client comes to the clinic complaining of a metallic taste in his mouth, blurred vision, tinnitus, and hand tremors. You question him about taking which of the following drugs?

   a. propranolol (Inderal)

   b. furosemide (Lasix)

   c. lithium carbonate (Eskalith)

   d. sertraline (Zoloft)

2. You are aware that your client has been depressed and is on medication. She has tachycardia and increased respirations, and she is sweating. You conclude that she is experiencing:

   a. a lithium overdose

   b. a TCA overdose

   c. an MAOI overdose

   d. an SSRI overdose

3. Lithium has been ordered for your client. You tell him that antimanic effects will take place in:

   a. 24 hours

   b. 3 days

   c. 5–7 days

   d. 10–14 days

4. Your client has been taking citalopram (Celexa). She is complaining of dizziness, nausea, and a headache. Before talking with her, you suspect that she has:

   a. increased her dosage to 40 mg daily

   b. either omitted doses or stopped taking the drug

   c. had a drug–drug interaction

   d. been smoking

5. Your client is taking isocarboxazid (Marplan). You caution her about eating:

   a. eggs

   b. aged cheeses

   c. onions

   d. strawberries

6. Your client is being treated for a mood disorder.

He is taking nefazodone (Serzone). You stress the importance of reporting to the physician which of the following?

   a. headache

   b. dizziness

   c. dark urine

   d. fatigue

7. Which of the following anticonvulsants is used in mood disorders?

   a. diazepam (Valium)

   b. phenytoin (Dilantin)

   c. lorazepam (Ativan)

   d. carbamazepine (Tegretol)

8. When a client appears depressed, the nurse should assess:

   a. suicidal thoughts

   b. blood pressure

   c. social skills

   d. habits

9. Your client comes to the clinic explaining that her husband wants her to stop taking fluoxetine (Prozac). Before you question her, you suspect that she is experiencing which adverse effect:

   a. headache

   b. dizziness

   c. sexual dysfunction

   d. heavy sedation

10. You are taking care of a 70-year-old woman who is depressed and is on an SSRI. Which of the following will you monitor over the next 3 months?

   a. smoking

   b. weight loss

   c. visual disturbances

   d. blood glucose levels

CHAPTER 11

Antiseizure Drugs

■ Exercises

Match the drug trade name to the generic name.

1. _____ levetiracetam

2. _____ clorazepate

3. _____ zonisamide

4. _____ valproic acid

5. _____ lorazepam

6. _____ phenytoin

7. _____ diazepam

8. _____ carbamazepine

9. _____ oxcarbazepine

10. _____ lamotrigine

a. Valium

b. Depakene (capsules)

c. Lamictal

d. Trileptal

e. Dilantin

f. Tegretol

g. Keppra

h. Ativan

i. Zonegran

j. Tranxene

Fill in the blank.

1. When more than one seizure occurs in a similar pattern, the disorder is called _____.

2. _____ is a common cause of seizures during late infancy and childhood.

3. _____ seizures start in a specific area of the brain.

4. _____ seizures are bilateral and symmetric, and have no defined point of origin.

5. The _____ phase of a seizure is characterized by rapid rhythmic and symmetric jerking movements of the body.

6. The _____ phase of a seizure is characterized by prolonged skeletal muscle contraction.

7. _____ seizures are defined as abrupt alterations in consciousness that last a few seconds.

8. _____ _____ is a life-threatening occurrence associated with tonic-clonic convulsions.

9. The most common adverse effects of phenytoin (Dilantin) affect the _____ and _____ _____.

10. _____ is the drug of choice for status epilepticus.

11. _____ should not be prescribed for children younger than 16 years of age because of a serious skin rash that may occur.

12. _____ is a newer drug given for partial seizures that inhibits abnormal neuronal firing but does not affect normal neuronal excitability.

13. _____ can be substituted for carbamazepine without tapering the dose.

14. The dosage of _____ should be reduced by one-half for a client with creatinine clearance below 70 mL/min.

15. _____ is used to treat bipolar disorders and to prevent migraine headaches.

16. _____ would not be prescribed for a client who is allergic to sulfonamides.

17. _____ reduces the effects of cardiovascular drugs.

18. Gingival hyperplasia often occurs in clients who take _____.

19. _____ and _____ decrease the effects of oral contraceptives and postmenopausal hormone replacement therapy.

20. _____ is the drug of choice for absence seizures.

■ Clinical Challenge

Your client has had his first seizure since he started taking carbamazepine 2 years ago. He experienced one seizure prior to drug therapy and has been on a dose of 400 mg bid since the seizure. He and his wife are extremely upset. They do not understand why he has had a seizure while on the medication. What assessment data would you obtain in order to respond to their concern?

■ Review Questions

1. In teaching your client the importance of taking her antiseizure drug at the same time each day, you explain that this will:
   a. decrease expected side effects of the drug
   b. help maintain therapeutic blood levels of the drug
   c. prevent further seizures
   d. make it easier for her to remember to take the medication

2. Your client has begun phenytoin (Dilantin) therapy. He asks you how long it will take for the drug to work. An appropriate response would be:
   a. "Approximately 7 to 10 days after phenytoin (Dilantin) is started, therapeutic blood levels should occur."
   b. "After a maximum of 3 weeks, benefits will be evident."
   c. "There is really no way to know how long it will take the drug to work."
   d. "There should be a decrease in seizure activity."

3. Topiramate (Topamax) is prescribed for your client. In your discussion about this drug with her, you would explain that:
   a. she should stop taking the drug if she experiences dizziness
   b. she can take the medication with or without food
   c. hypertension will occur
   d. she can take the drug with a full glass of water

4. One of the most common adverse effects of antiseizure medication is:
   a. diarrhea
   b. bradycardia
   c. drowsiness
   d. headaches

5. In assessing your client who is to start zonisamide (Zonegran) for generalized seizures, you should question him concerning:
   a. episodes of dizziness
   b. his diet
   c. a history of kidney stones
   d. chronic fatigue

6. In children 6 years and under, oral antiseizure drugs are rapidly absorbed and have short half-lives. This explains why:
   a. the rate of metabolism in children is decreased
   b. therapeutic blood levels are reached earlier in children than in adults
   c. children need lower doses of antiseizure drugs per kg of body weight than do adults
   d. excessive sedation is not a concern

7. A client is taking gabapentin (Neurontin). Which of the following lab tests should have been done before drug therapy was started?

   a. cholesterol

   b. partial thromboplastin time (PTT)

   c. creatinine clearance

   d. follicle stimulating hormone (FSH)

8. The most important goal for a client experiencing seizures is to:

   a. take medication as prescribed

   b. control seizure activity with minimal adverse drug effects

   c. avoid serious adverse drug effects

   d. keep follow-up appointments with health care provider

9. All of the following are true concerning antiseizure monotherapy in relation to combination drug therapy *except*:

   a. decreased compliance by the client

   b. fewer drug–drug interactions

   c. lower costs

   d. fewer adverse effects

10. Your assessment reveals that your client does not take his antiseizure medication as it is prescribed. He stated that not only did the medication make him "sleepy all the time," but it was also expensive. An appropriate nursing diagnosis would be:

    a. ineffective coping related to denial of seizure disorder

    b. deficient knowledge: drug effects

    c. noncompliance: inappropriate use of medication

    d. risk for injury: dizziness related to drug therapy

CHAPTER 12

Antiparkinson Drugs

■ Exercises

Match the following.

1. ____ dopamine

2. ____ levodopa/carbidopa (Sinemet)

3. ____ levodopa (Larodopa, Dopar)

4. ____ amantadine (Symmetrel)

5. ____ selegiline (Eldepryl)

6. ____ carbidopa (Lodosyn)

7. ____ tolcapone (Tasmar)

8. ____ entacopone (Comtan)

a. Antiviral agent used to increase dopamine levels

b. Increases dopamine in the brain by inhibiting its metabolism of monoamine oxidase (MAO)

c. Antiparkinson drug used to decrease the peripheral breakdown of levodopa

d. Ninety percent excreted through the biliary tract

e. Immediate release form of levodopa/carbidopa combination

f. Antiparkinson drug that is contraindicated in clients with liver disease

g. Most effective drug in treating Parkinson's disease

h. Neurotransmitter

Place T (true) or F (false) in each blank.

1. ____ Parkinson's disease occurs in both men and women between 50 and 80 years of age.

2. ____ People with Parkinson's disease have an increase in dopamine and a decrease in acetylcholine.

3. ____ Several drug combinations may be used before the start of levodopa therapy.

4. ____ Clients with Parkinson's disease may become depressed, isolated, and withdrawn.

5. ____ Iron increases absorption of levodopa.

6. ____ When dopaminergic drugs are discontinued, the dosage should be tapered over 1 week.

7. ____ The optimal dose of an antiparkinson drug is the largest one that allows the client to function.

8. ____ A dopamine agonist is given with levodopa/carbidopa to help relieve symptoms of Parkinson's disease.

9. ____ Levodopa becomes more effective after 5 to 7 years of use.

10. ____ Central activity anticholinergic drugs given for Parkinson's disease may cause confusion, agitation, and hallucinations.

Answer the following.

1. What causes Parkinson's disease?

2. Discuss the goal of antiparkinson drug therapy.

3. List two advantages of antiparkinson combination therapy.

4. What effect do antihistamines have on a client who is taking an anticholinergic drug for Parkinson's disease?

5. List side effects of levodopa.

■ Clinical Challenge

Your client asks you why she has developed dyskinesia. You are aware that she has been taking levodopa for several years. What would your response be? When she asks how long she will experience the involuntary movements of her tongue and mouth, what will you tell her?

■ Review Questions

1. Your client has been diagnosed with Parkinson's disease but is unable to take levodopa. Which of the following drugs may be used in her treatment plan?

    a. antipsychotic drugs

    b. anticholinergic drugs

    c. antiadrenergic drugs

    d. antiemetic drugs

2. When assessing a client who will probably be placed on levodopa, which of the following would the nurse be concerned about?

    a. narrow-angle glaucoma

    b. urinary retention

    c. dilated pupils

    d. hallucinations

3. To prevent or reduce nausea and vomiting, the nurse would encourage the client to take Sinemet:

    a. without regard to meals

    b. at bedtime

    c. during or right after a meal

    d. 2 hours prior to the noon meal

4. Your client is taking amantadine. Which of the following would be an appropriate nursing diagnosis?

    a. risk for injury: hypotension related to adverse effects of amantadine

    b. risk for injury: ataxia and dizziness related to adverse effects of antiparkinson drug

    c. alteration in nutrition: vomiting related to adverse effects of amantadine

    d. alteration in nutrition: anorexia related to adverse effects of an anticholinergic drug

5. You are working in a neuro clinic and see clients who have Parkinson's disease. When you observe clients who exhibit restlessness, agitation, and confusion, you suspect that:

    a. most are on levodopa/carbidopa combination drug therapy

    b. they are on levodopa therapy

    c. they are not taking the prescribed drugs

    d. they need to be reevaluated for drug therapy

6. Which of the following statements would indicate that the client understands levodopa therapy?

    a. "I will have to cut liver out of my diet."

    b. "If I don't feel better in 2 weeks, I will discontinue the levodopa."

    c. "I will take my medication at night."

    d. "I take an over-the-counter drug when I get a sinus infection."

7. Which instructions should the nurse give an older client who is taking benztropine (Cogentin)?

    a. "You must adhere to a strict low-sodium diet."

    b. "Avoid extreme heat and exercise."

    c. "Adverse effects will be greatly reduced if taken at night."

    d. "Diarrhea is a likely adverse effect."

8. Therapeutic effects of dopaminergic agents usually occur within:

    a. 24 hours

    b. 2 to 3 days

    c. 10 to 14 days

    d. 2 to 3 weeks

9. Your client is taking levodopa/carbidopa. Which of the following adverse effects is more likely to occur?

    a. hypertension

    b. constipation

    c. restlessness

    d. blurred vision

10. You are teaching your client about his new drug, pramipexole (Mirapex). You will stress that he should avoid which of the following?

    a. antihistamines

    b. alcohol

    c. antiemetics

    d. antipsychotics

CHAPTER 13

Skeletal Muscle Relaxants

■ Exercises

Answer the following.

1. Describe conditions that skeletal muscle relaxants are used to treat.

2. Discuss contraindications for the use of skeletal muscle relaxants.

3. What is the goal of treatment when skeletal muscle relaxants are used?

4. List common side effects of cyclobenzaprine (Flexeril).

5. Formulate two nursing diagnoses related to skeletal muscle relaxants.

Fill in the blank.

1. _____ is the only skeletal muscle relaxant that is not central acting.

2. _____ can cause physical dependence if used long term.

3. _____ is used to treat spasticity in spinal cord injuries and multiple sclerosis.

4. _____ is contraindicated in clients with recent myocardial infarctions.

5. _____ is contraindicated in clients with anemias.

6. _____ and _____ can be used to treat tetanus.

7. _____ is contraindicated in clients with prostatic hypertrophy.

8. _____ should not be used longer than 3 weeks.

9. _____ and _____ can cause liver damage.

10. _____ may potentially cause fatal hepatitis.

11. Abrupt withdrawal from _____ may cause hallucinations.

12. _____ may cause urine to turn green, brown, or black.

13. When administering IV _____, have the client lie down for at least 15 minutes after administration to avoid fainting.

14. _____ is used to treat malignant hyperthermia.

15. Baclofen, dantrolene, and _____ are used in chronic spastic disorders.

■ Clinical Challenge

Formulate three nursing diagnoses related to the use of dantrolene (Dantrium).

■ Review Questions

1. Your client is a 15-year-old male who has cerebral palsy. Which of the following skeletal muscle relaxants would he take for spasticity?
   a. orphenadrine (Norflex)
   b. methocarbamol (Robaxin)
   c. tizanidine (Zanaflex)
   d. metaxalone (Skelaxin)

2. Which of the statements by your client indicates that he has an understanding of methocarbamol (Robaxin) therapy?
   a. "I may develop a rash from this medication."
   b. "It takes at least 3 hours to feel the effects of my medication."
   c. "That drug is giving me diarrhea."
   d. "I would rather get my medication in an injection than take it by mouth."

3. Your client is experiencing muscle spasms from a four-wheeler accident. He is receiving 10 mg of cyclobenzaprine (Flexeril) tid. Your teaching plan should include which of the following instructions?
   a. Do not take the medication with food.
   b. Do not drive or operate heavy machinery for the first week.
   c. Increase the dosage if needed.
   d. Stop the drug if dizziness occurs.

4. A client is scheduled for surgery in the morning for a herniated spinal disk. He has been experiencing severe muscle spasms for the last 2 weeks. He will more than likely take which of the following skeletal muscle relaxants?
   a. metaxalone (Skelaxin)
   b. baclofen (Lioresal)
   c. dantrolene (Dantrium)
   d. tizanidine (Zanaflex)

5. Which of the following adverse effects may be significant for a client taking tizanidine (Zanaflex)?
   a. drowsiness
   b. dry mouth
   c. hypotension
   d. constipation

6. Which of the following clients would have the highest risk for hepatotoxicity from taking dantrolene (Dantrium) for 2 months?
   a. a 71-year-old female who is taking a cardiac glycoside and a diuretic
   b. a 53-year-old female who is on hormone replacement therapy
   c. a 22-year-old male who is taking a monoamine oxidase inhibitor
   d. a 56-year-old male who is receiving an antihypertensive agent

7. Which of the following is an adverse effect of cyclobenzaprine (Flexeril)?
   a. dry mouth
   b. bradycardia
   c. agitation
   d. insomnia

8. Your client has muscle spasms associated with multiple sclerosis. She is taking baclofen (Lioresal). At times, she needs help with activities. Her 10-year-old daughter has been helping her dress and comb her hair. However, your main concern is her drug therapy. An appropriate goal for the client would be:
   a. experience improved motor function
   b. take medication as prescribed
   c. experience relief from pain
   d. increase self-care in daily living activities

9. When a skeletal muscle relaxant is given for acute muscle spasms, which of the following would indicate a therapeutic effect?

   a. increased tenderness

   b. increased mobility

   c. decreased mobility

   d. decreased ability to maintain posture and balance

10. Your client is receiving dantrolene (Dantrium) 30 mg daily PO. Which of the following should be monitored periodically?

    a. prothrombin time and partial thromboplastin time

    b. urine specific gravity

    c. aspartate aminotransferase and alanine aminotransferase

    d. follicle stimulating hormone (FSH) levels

CHAPTER 14

Substance Abuse Disorders

■ Exercises

Define the following terms.

1. substance abuse

2. drug dependence

3. psychological dependence

4. physical dependence

5. tolerance

List withdrawal signs and symptoms of the following drugs or drug classifications.

1. barbiturates

2. alcohol

3. opiates

4. nicotine

Place T (true) or F (false) in each blank.

1. ____ Nurses can prevent abuse by promoting the use of nondrug measures when indicated.

2. ____ Volatile solvents are most often abused by men over the age of 40.

3. ____ Phencyclidine (PCP) produces intoxication similar to that of alcohol.

4. ____ It is difficult to predict the effects of marijuana.

5. ____ Mental alertness is associated with nicotine dependence.

6. ____ A person who abuses one drug will probably abuse others.

7. ____ Nicotine is the most abused drug in the world.

8. ____ Alcohol enhances the effects of hypoglycemia.

9. ____ Benzodiazepine agents are the drugs of choice for treating alcohol withdrawal syndrome.

10. ____ There is no antidote for barbiturate overdose.

Match the following.

1. ____ naltrexone (ReVia)

2. ____ acetone

3. ____ mescaline

4. ____ amphetamines

5. ____ flumazenil (Romazicon)

6. ____ heroin

7. ____ LSD

8. ____ "crack"

9. ____ dronabinol (Marinol)

10. ____ MDMA (3, 4 methylenedioxymethamphetamine)

a. Antidote for benzodiazepines
b. Referred to as "ecstasy"
c. Hallucinogen derived from lysergic acid
d. A legal cannabis preparation
e. A very potent, widely used form of cocaine
f. A volatile solvent
g. Used for narcolepsy
h. A semisynthetic derivative of morphine
i. Hallucinogen that is an alkaloid of the peyote cactus
j. Opiate antagonist

■ Clinical Challenge

You are on staff at a detoxification center. You are caring for a client who is experiencing barbiturate withdrawal. List signs and symptoms you will look for during the first 72 hours. What will the treatment of acute signs and symptoms involve? How long will your client need to be monitored for potential serious complications?

■ Review Questions

1. A client is admitted to the emergency room with multiple, non–life-threatening lacerations from a motor vehicle accident. You are aware that the accident was caused by alcohol ingestion. In obtaining a health history from a family member, you learn that he is on an anticoagulant. Which of the following should you observe for?

   a. decreased urinary output
   b. hypertension
   c. increased bleeding
   d. irritability

2. You work in a detoxification unit in a large hospital. You are assigned to work with clients experiencing alcohol withdrawal. Which of the following drugs would you use in the treatment of your clients?

   a. benzodiazepines
   b. monoamine oxidase inhibitors
   c. cardiac glycosides
   d. tetracyclines

3. Your client is receiving disulfiram (Antabuse) and complains of fatigue, headache, and dizziness. You explain that:

   a. you will ask the doctor to decrease the dose

   b. after about 2 weeks of treatment, the adverse effects usually subside.

   c. some people experience less pleasant adverse effects than he has

   d. the adverse effects will continue as long as he is taking the medication

4. Which of the following drugs would you administer to reduce symptoms of hyperactivity associated with alcohol withdrawal?

   a. lansoprazole (Prevacid)

   b. clonidine (Catapres)

   c. metyrose (Demser)

   d. triamcinolone (Aristocort)

5. Abuse of benzodiazepines can cause which of the following?

   a. seizures

   b. insomnia

   c. nightmares

   d. poor motor coordination

6. You are caring for a client who has abused a benzodiazepine for 5 years. She wants to stop taking the drug. Which of the following will you include when discussing withdrawal from this drug?

   a. Withdrawal symptoms usually begin 12 to 24 hours after the last dose.

   b. There will be no noticeable adverse effects.

   c. She may experience a seizure.

   d. She will be given methadone to help decrease withdrawal symptoms.

7. A client who has overdosed on a barbiturate is brought into the emergency room. The family reports that she has been unresponsive for 5 hours. After an artificial airway has been inserted, the nurse would:

   a. begin gastric lavage

   b. start IV fluids

   c. lower body temperature

   d. administer an emetic

8. You are caring for a client who abuses cocaine. Which of the following vital signs would you expect to find when assessing him?

   a. BP 98/50; P 120; R 40

   b. BP 130/88; P 92; R 28

   c. BP 150/90; P 80; R 16

   d. BP 170/98; P 110; R 20

9. Even though marijuana is illegal and not used for therapeutic purposes in the United States, it is useful in treating nausea and vomiting associated with anticancer drugs and in decreasing:

   a. intraocular pressure

   b. hypotension

   c. urinary output

   d. blood glucose levels

10. Assessment of an emergency room client reveals an elevated blood pressure, heart rate, and temperature; dilated pupils; and delusional thought processes. These symptoms indicate ingestion of:

    a. an opiate

    b. an amphetamine

    c. a hallucinogen

    d. a cannabinoid

CHAPTER 15

Central Nervous System Stimulants

■ Exercises

Fill in the blank.

1. _____ is a sleep disorder associated with "sleep attacks" during the day.

2. _____ increase norepinephrine, dopamine, and possibly serotonin in the brain.

3. Carbamazepine (Tegretol) can decrease the effects of _____.

4. _____ is the most common drug used in children for attention deficit-hyperactivity disorder (ADHD).

5. _____ given for narcolepsy may increase the effects of phenytoin (Dilantin).

6. _____ and sodium benzoate are sometimes used as a respiratory stimulant in neonates.

7. _____ is an over-the-counter drug used to promote wakefulness.

8. _____ is occasionally used as a respiratory stimulant.

9. _____ is contraindicated with a history of ventricular hypertrophy.

10. Central nervous system (CNS) stimulation is an adverse effect of _____.

List the following beverages according to the greatest amount of caffeine to the least amount of caffeine.

1. Iced tea

2. Espresso

3. Coke

4. Diet Pepsi

5. Mountain Dew

6. Mr. Pibb

7. Instant tea

Place a check in the appropriate box if the drug is used in narcolepsy and/or ADHD.

Drug	Narcolepsy	ADHD
Amphetamine		
Dexedrine		
Provigil		
Adderall		
Desoxyn		
Focalin		
Ritalin		

■ Clinical Challenge

Your client is a trial attorney who has narcolepsy. What potential problems do you see for him? Which drug might be prescribed to enable him to continue his profession? What is the expected outcome of drug therapy related to narcolepsy?

■ Review Questions

1. Your adult client is taking methylphenidate (Ritalin) for narcolepsy. He is to receive 40 mg bid. Which of the following times would be best for him to take his medication?

    a. 6 AM and 4 PM

    b. 8 AM and 8 PM

    c. 10 AM and 6 PM

    d. 10 PM and 6 AM

2. All of the following are considered desirable outcomes for clients who are taking CNS stimulants prescribed for narcolepsy except:

    a. balancing the checkbook

    b. raking leaves in the yard

    c. operating the lawnmower

    d. napping every day

3. In teaching a client who ingests several soft drinks a day to decrease caffeine intake, your instructions would be to avoid:

    a. Coke

    b. Mountain Dew

    c. Pepsi

    d. Dr. Pepper

4. Which of the following clients could safely use a CNS stimulant?

    a. a 38-year-old Caucasian female with glaucoma

    b. a 65-year-old African American male who experiences angina

    c. a 50-year-old male who has adult-onset diabetes

    d. a 28-year-old African American female with hyperthyroidism

5. A 6-year-old is taking methamphetamine (Desoxyn), 10 mg daily for ADHD. At each clinic visit, the nurse should assess:

    a. height and weight

    b. vision

    c. temperature

    d. blood pressure

6. A mother of a young client being treated for ADHD is concerned about her child having to take medication. An appropriate response to her would be:

    a. "The medication is needed to help your son function in society."

    b. "Without the medication, your son would not be able to go to school."

    c. "We can discuss the adverse effects of his medication if you like."

    d. "Hopefully, the medication can be omitted during the summer when he is out of school."

7. A client is being instructed on the use of modafinil (Provigil) for narcolepsy. Which of the following best reflects an expected goal of client-teaching activities related to the drug?

    a. Client will be able to identify two adverse effects of the drug.

    b. Family members will understand why the client must take the drug.

    c. Client will understand the physiological action of modafinil.

    d. Client will exercise three times a week.

8. Which of the following activities would the nurse be responsible for during the evaluation phase of drug therapy for a child receiving methylphenidate (Ritalin) for ADHD?

    a. preparation and administration of the drug

    b. ongoing monitoring of the child for therapeutic effects

    c. establishing outcome criteria related to the drug therapy

    d. gathering data related to a drug history

9. Counseling a mother concerning her 4-year-old daughter's treatment of ADHD would include the importance of:

    a. well-balanced meals

    b. increased physical activities

    c. limiting social encounters

    d. using sunscreen when outside

10. Which drug decreases the effects of modafinil (Provigil)?

    a. furosemide (Lasix)

    b. glipizide (Glucotrol)

    c. carbamazepine (Tegretol)

    d. buspirone (Buspar)

CHAPTER 16

Adrenergic Drugs

■Exercises

List five commonly used adrenergic drugs in each category.

Alpha and beta activity	Alpha activity	Beta activity

Match the following drugs with indications for their clinical use. Some may be used more than once; some may not be used at all.

1. ____ Tuamine

2. ____ Aramine

3. ____ Levophed

4. ____ Privine

5. ____ Ephedrine

6. ____ Neo-Synephrine

7. ____ Intropin

8. ____ Adrenalin

9. ____ Afrin

10. ____ Visine

a. Vasoconstriction in the eye

b. Gout

c. Cardiac stimulation

d. Hyperglycemia

e. Nasal decongestion

f. Ophthalmic conditions

g. Hypotension and shock

h. Hypertension

i. Diuresis

j. Bronchodilation

Place T (true) or F (false) in each blank.

1. ____ Ephedrine can be administered both orally and parenterally.

2. ____ Many over-the-counter preparations contain adrenergic drugs.

3. ____ Adrenergic drugs are given to decrease blood pressure.

4. ____ Antihistamines may decrease the effects of adrenergic drugs.

5. ____ Acute bronchospasm is most often relieved within 5 minutes of administration of epinephrine.

6. ____ You should not aspirate when giving epinephrine in a tuberculin syringe.

7. ____ The use of an adrenergic drug in a critically ill client may result in hyperglycemia.

8. ____ Epinephrine is the drug of choice to treat cardiac arrest.

9. ____ The most common use of epinephrine in children is for the treatment of asthma.

10. ____ Pseudoephedrine toxicity occurs with doses four to five times greater than the normal dose.

■ Clinical Challenge

Your client is to be given epinephrine for laryngeal edema associated with anaphylactic shock. How much epinephrine will you administer and in what type of syringe? What can the nurse do to accelerate relief of symptoms? How long should it take for the client to experience some relief?

■ Review Questions

1. When discussing nasal decongestants with a client in the allergy clinic, the nurse will impart information regarding:
   a. rebound congestion
   b. foods to be avoided
   c. compliance with allergy injections
   d. environmental factors

2. Your client is to have surgery and will have a general anesthetic. You will question her concerning the use of adrenergic drugs because of increased risk of:
   a. bronchial relaxation
   b. mydriasis
   c. cardiac dysrhythmias
   d. emotional disturbances

3. Which of the following drugs would be contraindicated for use with adrenergic drugs because of a potentially fatal outcome?
   a. Dopram
   b. Marplan
   c. Elavil
   d. Ritalin

4. Parenteral epinephrine may cause which of the following when administered to children?
   a. ataxia
   b. muscle twitching
   c. syncope
   d. excessive swallowing

5. Which route of administration is not used for epinephrine?
   a. inhalation
   b. injection
   c. oral
   d. topical

6. The client is experiencing a serious allergic reaction to a bee sting. Epinephrine is administered to relieve:
   a. pain and swelling around the sting site
   b. itching of skin around the site
   c. anxiety
   d. acute bronchospasm and laryngeal edema

7. A client has been taking pseudoephedrine (Sudafed) for nasal congestion. Which of the following adverse effects may he experience?
   a. bradycardia
   b. hypertension
   c. hypoglycemia
   d. hypothyroidism

8. You are to administer Sus-Phrine to your patient. Which of the following medication routes will you use?
   a. oral
   b. subcutaneous
   c. intramuscular
   d. intravenous

9. When teaching a client about the use of tetrahydrozoline hydrochloride (Visine), the nurse should advise which of the following?

   a. Wear a hat when outdoors.

   b. Drink a liter of fluid each day.

   c. Do not wear soft contact lenses while using the drug.

   d. Rest the eyes at least once every 2 to 3 hours.

10. The nurse has administered isoproterenol to a client who is in shock. An expected outcome would be which of the following?

   a. decreased pulse

   b. decreased blood pressure

   c. increased blood pressure

   d. increase in body temperature

CHAPTER 17

Antiadrenergic Drugs

■ Exercises

Answer the following.

1. Why are alpha$_1$ blocking agents used in benign prostatic hyperplasia (BPH)?

2. List five effects on the body caused by beta-adrenergic blocking agents.

3. What is the goal of antiadrenergic drug therapy?

4. Describe the blocking effects of antiadrenergic drugs.

5. What is the physiological action of alpha$_2$ agonist drugs?

Indicate the clinical use for each beta-adrenergic blocking agent by placing a check in the appropriate column.

Drug	Angina	Myocardial infarction	Tachydysrhythmia	Hypertension	Glaucoma
Atenolol					
Metoprolol					
Nadolol					
Propanolol					
Acebutolol					
Esmolol					
Sotalol					
Timolol					
Betaxolol					
Carteolol					
Levobunolol					
Metipranolol					

Match trade name of drug to generic name.

1. _____Catapres

2. _____Minipress

3. _____Dibenzyline

4. _____Cardura

5. _____Tenex

6. _____Wytensin

7. _____Flomax

8. _____Regitine

9. _____Priscoline

10. ____Aldomet

a. guanabenz

b. methyldopa

c. prazosin

d. tolazoline HCL

e. phentolamine

f. clonidine

g. doxazosin

h. phenoxybenzamine

i. guanfacine

j. tamsulosin

■ Clinical Challenge

A client is admitted to the hospital complaining of chest pains, palpitations, and shortness of breath. Blood pressure is 138/86, pulse is 94, and respirations are 24. After an extensive cardiac evaluation, she is sent home on propranolol (Inderal). Why was propranolol (Inderal) prescribed for this client? What information should the nurse tell the client about this drug? How long will the client take the drug?

■ Review Questions

1. The home health nurse is caring for a diabetic client who is taking metipranolol (OptiPranolol) for glaucoma. She will assess the client for:
   a. weight gain
   b. hypoglycemia
   c. headaches
   d. hyperglycemia

2. Clients who have received beta blockers after a myocardial infarction should be monitored for:
   a. hypertension and respiratory distress
   b. hypotension and heart failure
   c. hypertension and hyperthyroidism
   d. hyponatremia and kidney failure

3. Your client has cirrhosis and is taking tamsulosin (Flomax) for BPH. The nurse anticipates that the client will receive:
   a. a lower than usual dose of the drug
   b. twice as much as the usual dose
   c. a combination dose
   d. a normal adult dose

4. Early administration of a beta blocker after an acute myocardial infarction can decrease the occurrence of:
   a. renal failure
   b. heart block
   c. ventricular dysrrhythmias
   d. respiratory depression

5. Which of the following beta blockers is most frequently used in children?
   a. propranolol (Inderal)
   b. sotalol (Betapace)
   c. pindolol (Visken)
   d. nadolol (Corgard)

6. Your client is starting methyldopa (Aldomet) for hypertension. You would instruct the client to take the medication:
   a. on an empty stomach
   b. first thing in the morning
   c. with food
   d. at bedtime

7. An expected outcome for a client with benign prostatic hyperplasia who is on an alpha-blocking agent would be:

    a. increased blood pressure

    b. improved urination

    c. decreased blood glucose

    d. decreased sex drive

8. An adverse effect of propranolol that should be discussed with a client is:

    a. dizziness with activity

    b. excessive sleeping

    c. increased anxiety in crowds

    d. rapid weight loss

9. Your client is taking Aldomet. You would question her concerning her use of:

    a. steroids

    b. vitamins

    c. oral contraceptives

    d. sedatives

10. A client is leaving the hospital on a beta blocker. He has had a history of angina in the past but there are no major cardiac concerns at this time. Which of the following should he report to his physician?

    a. a weight gain of more than 2 pounds a week

    b. excessive energy

    c. a decreased appetite

    d. insomnia

■ Diagram

Fill in the blanks in Figure 17-1 with the terms below.

Epinephrine and norepinephrine
Beta adrenergic blocking drug
Nerve ending
Receptor site on cell surface
Myocardial or other tissue cell

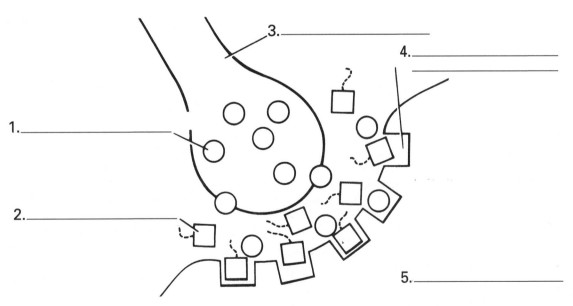

FIGURE 17-1.

CHAPTER 18

Cholinergic Drugs

■ Exercises

Fill in the blank.

1. Cholinergic drugs stimulate the _____ nervous system.

2. In myasthenia gravis, autoantibodies destroy _____ receptors for acetylcholine, which causes muscle weakness to occur.

3. The only therapeutic use for an irreversible anticholinesterase inhibitor is in the treatment of _____.

4. _____ is used to treat urinary retention due to urinary bladder atony.

5. _____, _____, and _____ are anticholinesterase agents approved for the treatment of Alzheimer's disease.

6. _____ is the prototype anticholinesterase agent.

7. _____ is used to differentiate between myasthenic and cholinergic crises.

8. _____ _____ is the only anticholinesterase that can cross the blood-brain barrier.

9. _____ is the maintenance drug of choice for clients with myasthenia gravis.

10. _____ can delay progression of Alzheimer's disease up to 55 weeks.

11. _____ is a drug used in the treatment of Alzheimer's disease that is metabolized by the liver and excreted in feces.

12. _____ is a centrally acting anticholinesterase agent that can cause hepatotoxicity.

13. _____ can be used in the neonate of a mother who has myasthenia gravis.

14. _____ can be used in severe cases of anticholinergic poisoning as an antidote.

15. _____ is a specific antidote to cholinergic agents.

Place T (true) or F (false) in each blank.

1. ____ Ingestion of clitocybe mushrooms causes cholinergic crises.

2. ____ All people who have myasthenia gravis require a caregiver to administer their medication.

3. ____ Myasthenia gravis is an autoimmune disorder.

4. ____ Cholinergic stimulation results in decreased peristalsis.

5. ____ Acetylcholine stimulates cholinergic receptors to promote normal urination.

6. ____ Direct-acting cholinergic drugs decrease respiratory secretions.

7. ____ Cholinergic drugs are contraindicated in peptic ulcer disease.

8. ____ Cholinergic drugs produce miosis.

9. ____ The best route for administration of bethanechol (Urecholine) is the oral route.

10. ____ Because of its duration of action, rivastigmine (Exelon) can be taken twice a day.

■ Clinical Challenge

A 52-year-old female has been diagnosed with myasthenia gravis. Her treatment plan includes pyridostigmine (Mestinon). Why would it be important to encourage the client or a family member to record symptoms associated with myasthenia gravis in relation to the effects of the drug therapy?

■ Review Questions

1. Your client has a confirmed diagnosis of myasthenia gravis and is started on pyridostigmine (Mestinon). The nurse is aware of the following adverse effect of pyridostigmine:

    a. dry mouth

    b. nausea

    c. constipation

    d. urinary retention

2. A 73-year-old man has been diagnosed with Alzheimer's disease and is started on tacrine (Cognex). Client instruction would include:

    a. Renal function should be monitored for 3 months.

    b. Cardiac enzymes should be monitored indefinitely.

    c. White blood cell count should be checked every month.

    d. Liver function should be monitored for at least 6 months.

3. It would be important to tell a client who has started on neostigmine (Prostigmin) that:

    a. he should limit fluids for a few days

    b. the drug could cause constipation

    c. he will take an oral form of the drug once a day for 5 days

    d. the drug acts within 1 hour of administration

4. The client, age 69, has a diagnosis of myasthenia gravis. She is experiencing abdominal cramping, diarrhea, weakness, and difficulty breathing. The nurse suspects cholinergic crisis and prepares which of the following?

    a. atropine 0.1 mg IV

    b. atropine 0.4 mg IM

    c. atropine 0.6 mg subq

    d. atropine 1.0 mg PO

5. A client's daughter calls the clinic and states that her mother, age 73, appears to be extremely dizzy. After questioning the daughter, you determine that the mother has Alzheimer's disease and is taking donepezil (Aricept). The nurse will be most concerned about the possibility of:

    a. headaches during the morning

    b. orthostatic hypotension

    c. injury while ambulating

    d. nausea and vomiting

6. You are working in a women's hospital where you are caring for a new mother who is experiencing postpartum urinary retention. Bethanechol (Urecholine) has been ordered. To prevent nausea and vomiting, you will administer the medication:

    a. before meals

    b. during meals

    c. after meals

    d. with a full glass of milk

7. Which of the following drugs decrease the effects of cholinergic agents?

    a. corticosteroids

    b. aminoglycoside antibiotics

    c. antihyperglycemics

    d. antihistamines

8. Your client has myasthenia gravis and is receiving pyridostigmine (Mestinon). She is complaining of nausea and vomiting. An appropriate response to her would be:

    a. "I'm so sorry, but that is to be expected."

    b. "Try taking your medication with food."

    c. "I'll talk to your doctor about decreasing the dose."

    d. "Make sure you get plenty of fluids during the day."

9. Parenteral bethanechol (Urecholine) is administered by which route:

   a. oral

   b. subcutaneous

   c. intramuscular

   d. intravenous

10. When neostigmine (Prostigmin) is given for postoperative distention, which of the following would indicate increased gastrointestinal muscle tone and motility?

    a. absence of flatus through the rectum

    b. increased urination

    c. presence of bowel sounds

    d. absence of bowel movements

CHAPTER 19

Anticholinergic Drugs

■Exercises

Match the following.

1. ____ ipratropium (Atrovent)

2. ____ trihexyphenidyl (Trihexy)

3. ____ benztropine (Cogentin)

4. ____ atropine

5. ____ flavoxate (Urispas)

6. ____ oxybutynin (Ditropan)

7. ____ tolterodine (Detrol)

8. ____ belladonna tincture

9. ____ scopolamine

10. ____ homatropine hydrobromide (Homapin)

a. Used in the treatment of parkinsonism and extrapyramidal reactions

b. Most often used for antispasmodic effects

c. Antimuscarinic, anticholinergic agent used to treat urinary frequency and urgency

d. Useful in treating rhinorrhea due to allergy or common cold

e. Increases bladder capacity

f. Useful in treating cystitis

g. Used to treat acute dystonic reactions

h. Prototype anticholinergic drug

i. Used for motion sickness

j. Ocular effects do not last as long as with atropine

Answer the following.

1. Describe the mechanism of action for anticholinergic drugs.

2. List five specific effects of anticholinergic drugs on the body.

3. Why are anticholinergic drugs given prior to surgery?

4. Why is atropine given with meperidine (Demerol) to relieve severe pain with renal colic?

5. List signs and symptoms of anticholinergic overdose.

6. How do tertiary amines and quaternary amines differ?

7. Why are oral anticholinergic drugs not given to treat asthma?

8. Why is the use of cyclopentolate (Cyclogyl) and tropicamide (Mydriacyl) guarded in children?

9. List five adverse effects associated with the use of anticholinergic drugs in the elderly.

10. Why do large doses of anticholinergic drugs cause facial flushing?

■ Clinical Challenge

Formulate three nursing diagnoses and a client goal for each in relation to anticholinergic drug therapy.

■ Review Questions

1. A client is being discharged from the hospital and will be taking dicyclomine (Bentyl) for irritable bowel syndrome. It will be important to instruct the client to:
   a. take the medication on an empty stomach
   b. limit intake of red meat
   c. take the drug 30 minutes before meals and at bedtime
   d. avoid drinking caffeinated beverages

2. You are a nurse in a large eye clinic and work in the client education department. You are working with a client who is receiving homatropine (Homapin). It is important to teach her:
   a. to stop the medication and call her physician if eye pain occurs
   b. that she cannot wear her contacts
   c. that she should rest her eyes two to three times a day
   d. that her visual acuity will decrease with use of the drug

3. Which of the following drugs can increase the effects of anticholinergic drugs?
   a. cardiac glycosides
   b. antihistamines
   c. anti-inflammatory agents
   d. oral hypoglycemics

4. Your client is 68 years old and is planning a cruise to Mexico. In anticipation of "sea sickness," he asks you for medication to prevent this. You suggest that his physician may prescribe a scopolamine patch but caution him concerning:
   a. heat stroke
   b. urinary retention
   c. decreased saliva
   d. diarrhea

5. Because of their adverse effect, urinary retention, anticholinergic drugs should not be prescribed for clients with:
   a. chronic constipation
   b. increased blood pressure
   c. prostatic hypertrophy
   d. urinary tract infections

6. Your client is planning a deep-sea fishing trip. He will take Transderm-V to protect him against motion sickness. You instruct him that a dose will provide protection for:
   a. 12 hours
   b. 24 hours
   c. 36 hours
   d. 72 hours

7. A client is receiving oxbutynin (Ditropan) for a neurogenic bladder. An expected outcome of this drug is:

   a. decreased frequency of voiding

   b. increased frequency of voiding

   c. decreased bladder capacity

   d. increased urgency in voiding

8. A client has been taking glycopyrrolate (Robinul) for adjunctive management of peptic ulcer disease for 3 years. The nurse questions him concerning:

   a. chronic diarrhea

   b. dental hygiene practices

   c. headaches

   d. diet

9. Anticholinergic drugs are contraindicated in which of the following?

   a. diabetes mellitus

   b. rheumatoid arthritis

   c. hyperthyroidism

   d. bradycardia

10. Your client has been taking propantheline bromide (Pro-Banthine) for irritable bowel syndrome. She tells you that the medication is making her constipated and confused at times. She states that she has missed a few doses because the "pills just cost too much." An appropriate nursing diagnosis for your client would be:

    a. constipation related to decrease in gastrointestinal motility

    b. disturbed thought process: confusion

    c. impaired urinary elimination: decreased bladder tone and urine retention

    d. noncompliance related to adverse drug effects and cost of the medication

CHAPTER 20

Hypothalamic, Pituitary, Parathyroid, and Adrenal Hormones

■ Exercises

Match the following.

1. _____ octreotide (Sandostatin)

2. _____ alendronate (Fosamax)

3. _____ calcitonin-human (Cibacalcin)

4. _____ aldosterone

5. _____ tamoxifen (Nolvadex)

6. _____ sodium chloride injection

7. _____ cosyntropin (Cortrosyn)

8. _____ raloxifene (Evista)

9. _____ lypressin

10. _____ calciferol

11. _____ calcitonin

12. _____ thyrotropin (Thytropar)

13. _____ teriparatide (Forteo)

14. _____ menotropins (Pergonal)

15. _____ oxytocin (Pitocin)

a. Used to test for suspected adrenal insufficiency

b. Lowers serum calcium in the presence of hypercalcemia

c. Used only for controlling excessive water of diabetes insipidus

d. Binds bone and inhibits calcium reabsorption from bone

e. Used in the treatment of Paget's disease

f. Treatment of choice for hypercalcemia

g. A fat soluble vitamin that functions as a hormone

h. A hypothalamic drug given for acromegaly

i. Used to prevent and treat breast cancer

j. A gonadotropin used to induce ovulation in the treatment of infertility

k. Main mineralocorticoid

l. Promotes uterine contractility and is used to induce labor and control post partum bleeding

m. A selective estrogen receptor modulator

n. Recommended for clients with severe osteoporosis

o. Used as a diagnostic agent to distinguish between primary and secondary hypothyroidism

Place T (true) or F (false) in each blank.

1. _____ Hormones may be given orally.

2. _____ Bisphosphonates must be taken with meals.

3. _____ Calcitonin-salmon helps to control pain in clients with osteoporosis.

4. _____ Most diets are throught to be deficient in calcium.

5. _____ Estrogen replacement therapy (ERT) is a treatment of choice for preventing postmenopausal osteoporosis.

6. _____ Excessive amounts of vitamin D can cause hypocalcemia.

7. _____ Hypocalcemia is common in children.

8. _____ Parathyroid hormone secretion is stimulated by low serum calcium levels.

9. _____ Pituitary hormones are given to replace or supplement naturally occurring hormones.

10. _____ There are many uses for hypothalamic and pituitary hormones.

■ Clinical Challenge

Your 65-year-old client has been told by her physician that she is at risk for osteoporosis. He has suggested that she begin alendronate (Fosamax). She asks you why she should take this medication. What would your response be? Which drugs would you question your client about that could predispose a woman to osteoporosis? What instructions would you give your client regarding alendronate (Fosamax)?

■ Review Questions

1. Your client, age 7, has a deficiency of endogenous growth hormone. She is started on somatropin (Humatrope) 0.03 mg/kg IM three times a week. Before the physician administers the first injection, you will check documentation for which of the following?

   a. evidence of open bone epiphyses

   b. daily urine output

   c. daily fluid input

   d. understanding of drug therapy

2. In teaching parents about growth hormone therapy for their child, the nurse will be sure to include:

   a. reporting the type of exercise the child participates in weekly

   b. monitoring the child's height and weight regularly

   c. recording the food intake daily

   d. administering the medication weekly

3. Hypocalcemia is the diagnosis for you client. Prior to drug therapy, you would expect his serum calcium level to be:

   a. below 8.5 mg/dL

   b. between 5.2 and 10 mg/dL

   c. above 12 mg/dL

   d. above 20 mg/dL

4. Your client is taking calcitriol (Rocaltrol) and is complaining of headaches, nausea, drowsiness, and muscle weakness. You suspect that she has:

   a. hypocalcemia

   b. hypercalcemia

   c. hypokalemia

   d. hyperkalemia

5. Which of the following would indicate that vasopressin is producing its therapeutic effect in your client?

   a. increased signs of dehydration

   b. decreased urine output

   c. decreased urine specific gravity

   d. increased thirst

6. Your client, age 9, has been taking somatrem (Protropin) for 3 years. On routine clinic visits, the nurse will monitor:

   a. blood pressure

   b. urine protein levels

   c. heart rate

   d. blood glucose levels

7. Which of the following is a common adverse effect of octreotide (Sandostatin)?

   a. nausea

   b. symptoms of gallstones

   c. hypoglycemia

   d. constipation

8. Which of the following would be an expected outcome for a client taking alendronate (Fosamax) for osteoporosis?

   a. decreased bone mass density

   b. presence of Chvostek's sign

   c. absence of bone fractures

   d. decreased serum calcium level

9. A client in the emergency room is being treated for hypercalcemia. The physician orders an injection of calcitonin (Calcimar). You are aware that the serum calcium level shoud decrease in:

a. 30 minutes

b. 1 hour

c. 2 hours

d. 3 hours

10. Which of the following should be included when instructing a client on how to take tetracycline and calcium preparations?

a. Take the drugs at the same time.

b. Take the drugs 2 to 3 hours apart.

c. Do not take calcium supplements when taking tetracycline.

d. Take the tetracycline 30 minutes after taking the calcium supplement.

CHAPTER 21

Thyroid and Antithyroid Drugs

■ Exercises

Fill in the blank.

1. Production of thyroxine and triiodothyronine depends on the presence of _____ and _____ in the thyroid gland.

2. _____ _____ is an enlargement of the thyroid gland resulting from iodine deficiency.

3. Synthetic _____ is the drug of choice in treating hypothyroidism.

4. Tyrosine is an amino acid derived from dietary _____.

5. _____ is the drug of choice for long-term treatment of hypothyroidism.

6. _____ drugs inhibit synthesis of thyroid hormones and do not damage the thyroid gland.

7. _____ preparations inhibit the release of thyroid hormones and cause them to be stored within the gland.

8. Levothyroxine is converted to _____ in peripheral tissues.

9. Serum _____ levels are used to monitor thyroid hormone replacement.

10. Thyroid hormones act by controlling _____ _____ _____.

Match the following.

1. ____ Synthroid

2. ____ Euthroid

3. ____ Propylthiouracil

4. ____ Cytomel

5. ____ Tapazole

6. ____ Lugol's solution

7. ____ Iodotope

8. ____ Inderal

9. ____ Lithium

10. ____ saturated solution of potassium iodide

a. Prototype of the thioamide antithyroid drugs

b. Used to treat short-term hyperthyroidism and as an expectorant

c. Used to treat symptoms of hyperthyroidism involving stimulation of the sympathetic nervous system

d. Synthetic preparation of T_3

e. Acts synergistically with antithyroid drugs to produce hypothyroidism

f. Drug of choice for long-term treatment of hypothyroidism

g. Used to treat thyroid cancer

h. Similar to propylthiouracil (PTU), is well absorbed and reaches peak plasma levels quickly

i. Used to treat thyrotoxic crisis

j. Similar to composition of natural thyroid hormone

Place T (true) or F (false) in each blank.

1. ____ Thyroxine is more potent than triiodothyronine.

2. ____ The thyroid gland extracts iodine from the circulating blood.

3. ____ The thyroid-stimulating hormone (TSH) stimulates the thyroid gland to release thyroid hormones into circulation.

4. ____ Iodine preparations are used alone in the treatment of hyperthyroidism.

5. ____ Hypothyroidism and hyperthyroidism produce opposing effects on the body.

6. ____ To compensate for decreased production of thyroid hormone, the anterior pituitary gland secretes less TSH.

7. ____ Simple goiter is common in the United States.

8. ____ Iodine preparations reduce serum levels of thyroid hormones more quickly than do thioamide drugs.

9. ____ Taking levothyroxine on an empty stomach decreases absorption of the drug.

10. ____ Thyroid replacement therapy in clients with hypothyroidism is lifelong.

■ Clinical Challenge

Your client, a 42-year-old female, has been diagnosed with hypothyroidism. She is placed on Synthroid 0.05 mg/day PO. She is concerned that her dose may have to be increased. What do you tell her in response to her concern? What will be included in your teaching plan for her?

■ Review Questions

1. Which of the following is an initial indication that your client has primary hypothyroidism?
   a. serum TSH of 5.2 microunits/L
   b. serum TSH of 0.1 microunits/L
   c. serum TSH of 0.5 microunits/L
   d. serum TSH of 3 microunits/L

2. Your client has been diagnosed with hyperthyroidism. You expect that an appropriate nursing diagnosis related to her weight would be:
   a. imbalanced nutrition: less than body requirements
   b. imbalanced nutrition: more than body requirements
   c. swallowing: impaired
   d. oral mucous membranes: altered

3. An expected outcome for your patient who has been on thyroid medication would be:
   a. decreased pulse rate
   b. increased blood pressure
   c. increased energy and activity levels
   d. decreased appetite

4. Your client has been recently started on levothyroxine (Synthroid). All of the following would be included in the teaching plan *except*:
   a. Never take over-the-counter drugs unless the physician has been consulted.
   b. Avoid the herb ephedra.
   c. Synthroid may be switched to Levothroid.
   d. Limit intake of caffeine beverages to two or three a day.

5. Your client is taking levothyroxine (Levothroid) and explains to you that occasionally he has to take an antacid for heartburn. Your best response to him would be:
   a. "Take the two medications together."
   b. "You should not take an antacid when taking Levothroid."
   c. "Take your thyroid medication 2 hours before you take the antacid."
   d. "Skip the Levothroid dose when you take the antacid."

6. Your client, age 28, has primary hypothyroidism and is taking liotrix (Euthroid). She asks you how long she will have to take the medication. Your response to her would be:

   a. "Just for a few weeks."

   b. "You will take the medication for 1 year, then your physician will taper your dose for a few months."

   c. "Usually, people with hypothyroidism will need to take their medication for the rest of their lives."

   d. "Don't worry about that now. We will discuss it later."

7. Your client is 25 years old and is on thyroid hormone replacement. She is also taking an oral contraceptive. You suspect that her thyroid medication will need to be:

   a. increased

   b. decreased

   c. kept the same

   d. discontinued

8. Propranolol (Inderal) is given to your client who has been diagnosed with hyperthyroidism. This drug:

   a. enhances the effects of PTU

   b. controls symptoms resulting from excessive stimulation of the sympathetic nervous system

   c. converts levothyroxine hormone to liothyronine (T_3).

   d. replaces the thyroid hormone from an exogenous source.

9. Your client has been placed on PTU. Your assessment data reveal that he is on digoxin. You expect the physician to:

   a. discontinue the digoxin

   b. increase the dosage of digoxin

   c. keep the dosage of the digoxin the same

   d. reduce the dosage of digoxin

10. Your client is taking PTU for hyperthyroidism. Which of the following instructions should be given to him concerning administration of his medication?

   a. Take the medication every 8 hours around the clock.

   b. Take the medication once daily.

   c. If a dose is missed, double the next dose.

   d. Take the daily dose at bedtime.

CHAPTER 22

Antidiabetic Drugs

■ Exercises

Match the following.

1. ____ sulfonylureas

2. ____ oral antidiabetic drugs

3. ____ hypoglycemia

4. ____ glycogenolysis

5. ____ insulin

6. ____ alpha-glucosidase inhibitors

7. ____ hyperglycemia

8. ____ ketoacidosis

9. ____ meglitinide

10. ____ glucose

a. Increased appetite

b. Dosage is flexible and depends on food intake

c. Some of these drugs can lower blood sugar by decreasing absorption or production of glucose

d. Blood glucose below 60 to 70 mg/dL

e. Oldest and largest group of oral antidiabetic drugs

f. A life-threatening complication that occurs with severe insulin deficiency

g. Breakdown of glycogen

h. A protein hormone secreted by beta cells in the pancreas

i. Characterized by excessive thirst, hunger, and increased urine output

j. Delays digestion of complex carbohydrates into glucose and simple sugars.

Place T (true) or F (false) in each blank.

1. ____ Insulin is the only drug used to treat type 1 diabetes.

2. ____ Insulin is never given to clients with type 2 diabetes.

3. ____ Insulin is contraindicated in hypoglycemia.

4. ____ Insulin can be given orally.

5. ____ Insulin that has been refrigerated should be used within 1 year.

6. ____ Metformin is often the initial drug of choice in obese clients with newly diagnosed type 2 diabetes.

7. ____ Glitazones are contraindicated in clients with liver disease.

8. ____ Ginseng increases blood glucose levels.

9. ____ Dosage of insulin must be individualized according to blood glucose levels.

10. ____ Insulin can be given with all types of oral antidiabetic drugs.

11. ____ Clients with diabetic ketoacidosis have an increase of insulin in the body.

12. ____ There are higher levels of insulin in clients with hepatic impairment because less insulin is metabolized.

13. ____ Insulin is absorbed faster from the upper arm than the abdomen.

14. ____ Sulfonylureas lower bood glucose by decreasing secretion of insulin.

15. ____ Symptoms of hypoglycemia are excess thirst, hunger, and increased urine output.

16. ____ Symptoms of hyperglycemia include sweating, nervousness, weakness, tremors, and mental confusion.

17. ____ Glucosamine is harmful to people with diabetes.

18. ____ The liver is important in restoring blood sugar levels.

19. ____ Alcohol decreases the effects of metformin.

20. ____ Omitting or decreasing insulin dosage may lead to ketoacidosis.

Complete the chart for the different types of insulin.

Type	Onset	Peak	Duration
Regular Iletin II			
NPH			
Humalog			
Humulin N			
Ultralente			
Novolin R			

▪ Clinical Challenge

Your client is a 48-year-old Native American. She has been diagnosed with type 2 diabetes. She is 50 pounds overweight and has known allergies to sulfa drugs. Which oral antidiabetic drug will she most likely be started on? What information will be considered in the selection of her medication?

▪ Review Questions

1. You are teaching a mother of a newly diagnosed diabetic child how to assess for hypoglycemia. Which of the following signs will you include?

   a. increased urine output
   b. increased hunger
   c. shakiness/nervousness
   d. excessive thirst

2. Before a client is started on metformin (Glucophage), he should be assessed for which of the following?

   a. renal disease
   b. anemia
   c. osteoporosis
   d. hypertension

3. Your client has been controlled on 30 U of NPH insulin for several years. Recently, he was placed on prednisone for rheumatoid arthritis. You suspect that, due to the prednisone therapy, the NPH dosage may:

   a. stay the same

   b. need to be increased

   c. be discontinued for a short period

   d. need to be decreased

4. A client who takes NPH insulin asks you about the use of an insulin pump. In considering her question, you are aware that which of the following insulins is used in a pump?

   a. NPH

   b. Ultralente

   c. Lente

   d. Regular

5. A 38-year-old client is receiving 30 U of NPH insulin and 8 U of regular insulin at 7:30 AM. She is receiving 25 U of NPH insulin and 5 U of regular insulin at 3:30 PM. Her blood glucose levels have been elevated by 10:30 AM for the last several days. What adjustments should be made in her insulin therapy?

   a. Both morning doses of NPH and regular insulin should be increased.

   b. The morning dose of regular insulin should be increased.

   c. Both afternoon doses should be increased.

   d. The afternoon NPH dose should be increased.

6. A client receives 25 units of NPH insulin at 8 AM. At what time of day should the nurse be alert for a potential hypoglycemic reaction?

   a. after breakfast

   b. before breakfast

   c. at bedtime

   d. before dinner (evening meal)

7. Your client has been on metformin (Glucophage) for 5 years. He is scheduled for major surgery in 2 weeks. You inform him that:

   a. his metformin dose will increase

   b. he will be taken off of metformin and placed on insulin therapy during surgery and for some time after surgery

   c. he will take metformin as prescribed during and after surgery

   d. he will not need to take therapy for diabetes during or after surgery

8. Your client will be taking insulin lispro (Humalog). What instructions do you need to give to him concerning the administration of this drug?

   a. Take 1 hour before meals.

   b. Take at bedtime only.

   c. Take 1½ hours after meals.

   d. Take 15 minutes prior to meals.

9. Your client has just been diagnosed with type 1 diabetes and is placed on regular and NPH insulin. When teaching her about self-administration of her medication, you will most likely advise her to:

   a. administer medications separately in two syringes

   b. administer both medications in one syringe, drawing up the regular insulin first

   c. administer the regular insulin first, then check the blood sugar to determine whether NPH is needed

   d. administer both medications together, drawing up the NPH insulin first

10. Which of the following statements from your client indicates a need for further education regarding diabetes therapy?

    a. "I will need more insulin on the days I take my aerobics class."

    b. "I wear a medical alert bracelet at all times stating that I am diabetic."

    c. "I get a family member to check my syringe and make sure I have drawn up the correct dose of insulin."

    d. "I know that I should eat my meals at regularly scheduled times."

CHAPTER 23

Drug Use During Pregnancy and Lactation

■ Exercises

Place a T (true) or F (false) in each blank.

1. ____ Many drugs are considered safe during pregnancy.

2. ____ Drug effects are more predictable during pregnancy than when in the nonpregnant state.

3. ____ In the fetus, a large proportion of a drug dose is active because the fetus has low levels of serum albumin and low levels of drug binding.

4. ____ Drug teratogenicity is most likely to occur during the first trimester of pregnancy.

5. ____ Small amounts of alcohol during pregnancy are considered safe.

6. ____ Caffeine is the most commonly ingested drug during pregnancy.

7. ____ Cigarette smoking during pregnancy can cause fetal and infant death.

8. ____ Marijuana can cause third-trimester bleeding.

9. ____ Abruptio placentae can occur from ingestion of cocaine during the third trimester of pregnancy.

10. ____ Herbal supplements are recommended during pregnancy.

11. ____ Human insulin may be needed during gestational diabetes.

12. ____ Amoxicillin may be used to treat a urinary tract infection during pregnancy.

13. ____ Women who are insulin dependent are more likely to need smaller doses during pregnancy.

14. ____ Methyldopa is the drug of choice for the pregnant hypertensive woman.

15. ____ Women with epilepsy should double their routine dose of folic acid during pregnancy.

Match the following.

1. ____ ferrous sulfate

2. ____ magnesium sulfate

3. ____ meclizine (Antivert)

4. ____ aspirin

5. ____ ritodrine (Yutopar)

6. ____ oxytocin (Pitocin)

7. ____ folic acid

8. ____ methylergonovine (Methergine)

9. ____ meperidine (Demerol)

10. ____ Metamucil

a. Used to treat anemia during pregnancy

b. May be used for prophylaxis in women at risk of developing preeclampsia

c. Used to treat nausea and vomiting during pregnancy

d. Drug of choice used to prevent or treat seizures during preeclampsia and eclampsia

e. Stimulates uterine contractions to initiate labor

f. Narcotic analgesic used during labor and delivery

g. May be used during pregnancy for constipation

h. Used in the management of postpartum hemor-rhage

i. Relaxes uterine smooth muscle, which will slow or stop uterine contractions

j. Necessary to prevent neural tube birth defects

■ Clinical Challenge

Your client is a 28-year-old who is 30 weeks pregnant and has diabetes mellitus. She is insulin dependent and is being followed closely by a home health nurse. The client presents with signs of preterm labor in the emergency department. She is admitted and started on IV ritodrine (Yutopar). How will you prepare ritodrine for administration? How long will the client receive this medication?

In order to facilitate uterine placental blood flow, how should the client be positioned during the administration of the medication?

Uterine suppression is successful, and the client is to be discharged on an oral dosage of ritodrine. What instructions do you give to the client?

■ Review Questions

1. Your client is 20 weeks pregnant, and fetal heart tones can no longer be heard. It is determined that the pregnancy is to be terminated. Which of the following drugs will be given after mifepris-tone to make sure of full expulsion of the con-ceptus?

   a. ritodrine

   b. prostaglandin

   c. methylergonovine

   d. oxytocin

2. Your client is receiving a tocolytic. Which of the following may indicate hypermagnesemia?

   a. increased blood pressure of 170/90

   b. decreased heart rate of 60

   c. decreased respiratory rate of 8

   d. increased body temperature of 102°

3. Which of the following indicates an appropriate dose of vitamin K for a neonate at delivery?

   a. 0.25 to 0.5 mg

   b. 0.5 to 1 mg

   c. 1 to 1.5 mg

   d. 2.5 to 5 mg

4. You are counseling a group of pregnant women at the health department concerning use of immunizations during pregnancy. You should stress that which of the following immunizations should not be taken during pregnancy?

   a. influenza

   b. rubella

   c. hepatitis B

   d. tetanus

5. Oxytocin is the drug of choice for prevention and control of postpartum uterine hemorrhage because it is unlikely to cause:

   a. hypotension

   b. hypertension

   c. tachycardia

   d. bradycardia

6. In order to decrease the risk of hypotension while receiving IV ritodrine (Yutopar) the client should be placed in which of the following positions?

    a. prone

    b. supine

    c. side-lying

    d. semi-Fowler's

7. Which of the following drugs should be completely avoided during pregnancy?

    a. nicotine

    b. caffeine

    c. acetaminophen

    d. alcohol

8. Tetracyclines are contraindicated during pregnancy because they:

    a. decrease the white blood cell count in the mother

    b. interfere with the development of teeth and bone in the fetus

    c. interfere with folic acid metabolism in the fetus

    d. cause long bone growth retardation in the fetus

9. A 40-year-old has just been told by her health care provider that she is pregnant. She has a history of mild hypertension and is concerned about taking medication during pregnancy. An appropriate response should include:

    a. "Hydralazine is considered safe to use during pregnancy."

    b. "Guanfacine can be used in reduced dosages."

    c. "All antihypertensive drugs are unsafe to use during pregnancy."

    d. "Diuretics can be given during pregnancy to treat hypertension."

10. Which of the following drugs is used to promote fetal production of surfactant?

    a. furosemide

    b. ergotamine

    c. nifedipine

    d. betamethasone

CHAPTER 24

Drugs Affecting Female Reproductive Health

■ Exercises

Place T (true) or F (false) in each blank.

1. ____ Estrogens and progestins are synthesized from cholesterol.

2. ____ Small amounts of estrogens are found in adipose tissue.

3. ____ Estrone is the major estrogen.

4. ____ During pregnancy, the placenta produces small amounts of estriol.

5. ____ When fertilization does not take place, levels of estrogen and progesterone increase.

6. ____ If an ovum is fertilized, progesterone acts to maintain the pregnancy.

7. ____ Most hormonal contraceptives are synthetic estrogen and progestin.

8. ____ Decreased pituitary stimulation of the ovaries may result in the need for estrogen replacement therapy.

9. ____ Women who take hormones should have a complete physical every 3 years.

10. ____ Oral contraceptives increase the effects of insulin.

Answer the following.

1. Describe the main function of estrogen.

2. Why is progestin used in hormone replacement therapy?

3. List five contraindications to hormone therapy.

4. Describe the three mechanisms of hormonal contraception.

Fill in the blank.

1. _____ is secreted by the corpus luteum during the last half of the menstrual cycle.

2. Estrogens are inactivated in the _____.

3. During pregnancy, increased levels of _____ cause the uterus and breast to enlarge and relaxation of the ligaments and joints in the pelvis.

4. _____ prepares the breasts for lactation by promoting development of milk-producing cells.

5. The most widely used synthetic steroid estrogen is _____ _____.

6. _____ _____ is an herb used to treat symptoms of menopause.

7. _____ is the only drug approved by the FDA for postcoital contraception.

8. _____ is used as a transdermal patch that releases slowly into the vascular system.

9. _____ is a drug used that is identical to human gonadotropin hormone (GnRH) and is used to treat infertility.

10. _____ is used for excessive prolactin levels to correct amenorrhea and infertility.

■ Clinical Challenge

Your client, age 48, comes to the health clinic with symptoms of postmenopausal syndrome. She complains of fatigue, hot flashes, and increased perspirations. What assessment data will you obtain from the client? Your client is placed on hormone replacement therapy. Outline a teaching plan for her.

■ Review Questions

1. A 19-year-old female is seen in the clinic for unprotected sexual intercourse the night before. She is requesting emergency contraception. Which of the following drugs will she be given?
   a. Estraderm
   b. Prempro
   c. Preven
   d. Cenestin

2. Your client has been placed on hormone replacement therapy. Provera has been prescribed for her. She should be instructed that she is at risk for:
   a. colon cancer
   b. gall bladder disease
   c. Alzheimer's disease
   d. osteoporosis

3. A client who has been placed on estrogen complains of nausea. The nurse should instruct her to:
   a. eat six small meals a day
   b. take her medication before breakfast
   c. drink a full glass of water with each pill
   d. take medication after meals or at bedtime

4. Your client will be using estradiol skin patches for hormone replacement therapy. You teach her that she should apply the patch:
   a. to the abdomen
   b. to her breast
   c. in the waistline area
   d. on the forearm

5. Your client has a history of seizures and is taking carbamazepine. Her physician has just prescribed an oral contraceptive for her. The client will be informed that she should:
   a. use an additional birth control method
   b. stop taking her seizure medication
   c. ask her neurologist about decreasing her dose of carbamazepine
   d. take her seizure medication at night with her oral contraceptive

6. A client has been placed on Premarin 1 mg daily. The nurse will advise which of the following in her teaching session with the client:
   a. Take the medication only when needed.
   b. Report to the emergency room if nausea occurs.
   c. Avoid exercise.
   d. Monitor her weight.

7. You are assessing a client who will be placed on hormone replacement therapy. Which of the following data would cause immediate concern?
   a. walking 2 miles a day
   b. cigarette smoking
   c. eating large meals
   d. occasional headaches

8. A client has requested to be placed on hormone replacement therapy for severe hot flashes and fatigue. She has been told that she is not a good candidate for hormone replacement therapy. You suspect she has a history of:

   a. kidney disease

   b. thromboembolic disease

   c. asthma

   d. osteoporosis

9. Your client has been taking birth control pills for 3 years. She calls the clinic to tell you that she has had a stomach virus and has been unable to take her pills for 2 days. Which of the following responses would be appropriate?

   a. "Take three pills today and continue as prescribed."

   b. "Take two pills now!"

   c. "You need to speak to your physician."

   d. "Take two pills today and two tomorrow, then continue as prescribed."

10. Which of the following would the nurse encourage a patient to report if taking an oral contraceptive?

   a. headaches

   b. calf tenderness

   c. weight loss

   d. nausea

CHAPTER 25

Drugs Affecting Male Reproductive Health

■ Exercises

Answer the following.

1. Name three organs of the body that secrete androgens.

2. List the three functions of testosterone.

3. Why are androgens and anabolic steroids classified as Schedule III drugs?

4. List 10 potentially serious side effects of anabolic steroids.

Fill in the blank.

1. Male sex hormones are synthesized from _____.

2. Androgens produced by the ovaries are used as precursor substances for the production of naturally occurring _____.

3. _____ is the only important male sex hormone.

4. _____ is a transdermal form of testosterone that has a rapid onset of action and lasts approximately 24 hours.

5. Testoderm must be applied to the _____ to achieve adequate blood levels.

6. _____ may be used to prevent or treat endometriosis or fibrocystic breast disease in women.

7. _____ inhibits the metabolism of carbamazepine and increases risks of toxicity.

8. Androgens and anabolic steroids are contraindicated in clients with preexisting _____ disease.

9. Testosterone is secreted by _____ cells in the testes in response to stimulation by the luteinizing hormone from the anterior pituitary gland.

10. Testosterone increases the formation of _____ throughout the body.

■ Clinical Challenge

You and your spouse are at a social gathering. Someone asks you what you think of the rumor going around town about the high school football team and anabolic steroids. What would your response be?

■ Review Questions

1. Your client has acquired primary hypogonadism and is to begin testosterone therapy. Testoderm has been prescribed. He is instructed to apply the patch to his:
   a. forearm
   b. scrotum
   c. buttocks
   d. upper back

2. A client is to start testosterone therapy. Testoderm TTS has been prescribed. The health care provider instructs him to change the patch:
   a. every 12 hours
   b. daily
   c. every 3 days
   d. weekly

3. A 62-year-old is on androgen therapy. The nurse will inform him of which of the following possible adverse effects?
   a. increased sperm count
   b. increased libido
   c. high-pitched voice
   d. increased pubic hair

4. A 13-year-old client takes testosterone because his father had delayed puberty. The client will be assessed for which of the following every 6 months?
   a. migraine headaches
   b. altered long bone growth
   c. hyperglycemia
   d. increased hair growth

5. You work in a women's clinic. You are aware that women who are unresponsive to conventional therapy for endometriosis are given which of the following?
   a. danazol (Danocrine)
   b. testosterone enanthate (Delatestryl)
   c. testosterone cypionate (Depo-Testosterone)
   d. methyltestosterone (Methitest)

6. Your client, age 48, is taking testosterone for hypogonadism due to an androgen deficiency. Which of the following lab tests should be done during therapy?
   a. lipid levels
   b. cardiac enzymes
   c. sperm count levels
   d. hepatic function levels

7. Your client, age 15, is taking testosterone. You suspect he is concerned about his appearance. Which of the following nursing diagnoses would be appropriate for him?
   a. disturbed self-esteem
   b. disturbed personal identity
   c. deficient knowledge
   d. ineffective sexuality patterns

8. A 58-year-old male is requesting sildenafil (Viagra). The nurse will question him concerning which of the following?
   a. sexual activity
   b. exercise tolerance
   c. eating habits
   d. use of nitrates

9. Alprostadil is used to manage:
   a. hypogonadism
   b. endometriosis
   c. body building
   d. erectile dysfunction

10. A 56-year-old female has been placed on testolactone (Teslac) for breast cancer. Which of the following will likely be a concern for her?
    a. high blood pressure
    b. increase in appetite
    c. excessive growth of hair
    d. headaches

CHAPTER 26

Nutritional Support Products

■ Exercises

Match the following.

1. ____ pancreatin (Creon)

2. ____ Isocal

3. ____ Prosobee

4. ____ MCT Oil

5. ____ Nepro

6. ____ Amin-Aid

7. ____ Lofenalac

8. ____ Nutrivent

9. ____ Pregestimil

10. ____ Enfamil

a. A preparation used in adults with fat malabsorption syndromes

b. An enteral product for clients with chronic obstructive pulmonary disease

c. A formula used in infants and children with phenylketonuria

d. Milk substitute given to infants who are allergic to milk

e. Preparation of pancreatic enzymes used to aid in digestion

f. A formula used in infants with severe malabsorption disorders

g. An infant formula similar to human breast milk

h. A high-calorie, low-electrolyte enteral formulation

i. A nutritional supplement that is isotonic and should be given full strength

j. A source of protein for clients with acute or chronic renal failure

Place T (true) or F (false) in each blank.

1. ____ The safest and most effective way of replacing body fluids is to give oral fluids.

2. ____ An indication of water deficit is drowsiness.

3. ____ When oral feedings are contraindicated but the gastrointestinal tract is functioning, IV fluids are preferred over tube feedings.

4. ____ Carbohydrates and fats serve as sources of energy for cellular metabolism.

5. ____ A fat emulsion can supply more calories to a client than an IV solution of dextrose and protein.

6. ____ Tube feedings are usually initiated with small amounts of diluted solution and then increased to larger amounts and full strength solution.

7. ____ Parenteral feedings are indicated when the gastrointestinal tract is nonfunctioning.

8. ____ An IV solution should contain at least 20% dextrose.

9. ____ An IV solution is nutritionally adequate.

10. ____ Antacids may increase the effects of pancreatic enzymes.

▪ Clinical Challenge

A 56-year-old female with recurring colon cancer is recovering from extensive surgery involving the colon, right kidney, the bladder, right fallopian tube, and the uterus. She is sent home 10 days postoperatively. After 4 days of being at home, her husband calls her physician and tells him that she cannot eat, has lost 8 pounds, and is lethargic. She is readmitted into the hospital and started on parenteral feedings. Why is the client receiving parenteral feedings? The husband asks how long she will receive the parenteral feedings. What will your response be?

The physician discharges the client after 5 days of hospitalization, and she is to continue the feedings at home. What will be your instructions?

▪ Review Questions

1. You are caring for a client who has chronic renal failure and is receiving dialysis. Which of the following nutritional supplements may be ordered for him?

   a. Liposyn

   b. Nepro

   c. Pulmocare

   d. Suplena

2. For an intermittent tube feeding, which of the following is considered the appropriate administration time?

   a. 5 to 10 minutes

   b. 15 to 20 minutes

   c. 30 to 60 minutes

   d. 60 to 90 minutes

3. Your client comes to the clinic complaining about the "bad" taste of MCT oil. She indicates that she is going to stop drinking the preparation. Your response to her should be:

   a. "I'll talk to your doctor and see whether we can change your enteral preparation."

   b. "Mix it with water and drink it as fast as you can."

   c. "You may mix this preparation with your favorite fruit juice."

   d. "I know. It tastes terrible. I would stop taking it, too."

4. You are in charge of orientation for new RN graduates who are working in a long-term care facility. When instructing them concerning intermittent tube feedings, you will advise that:

   a. tubing should be changed every 24 hours

   b. tube placement does not have to be checked before feeding

   c. solutions should be heated prior to use

   d. administration should be over a 10-minute period

5. A major complication of tube feeding is:

   a. aspiration of formula into the lungs

   b. irritation of the esophagus

   c. pancreatitis

   d. diarrhea

6. Your client is receiving an intravenous fat emulsion. Which of the following lab values should be checked before administration?

   a. blood glucose levels

   b. serum sodium levels

   c. triglyceride levels

   d. potassium levels

7. Increasing calorie intake for your client who has chronic obstructive pulmonary disease may lead to:

   a. increased carbon dioxide production

   b. decreased carbon dioxide production

   c. decreased need for oxygen

   d. respiratory alkalosis

8. A 78-year-old is admitted to the emergency room with a complaint of excessive vomiting and diarrhea for 6 days. You will note the following signs of water deficit *except*:

a. increased hematocrit

b. flushed skin

c. drowsiness

d. dry mucous membranes

9. Your client is to begin taking pancrelipase (Viokase). Instructions regarding administration should include taking the medication:

a. at least 2 hours prior to eating

b. immediately before or with meals

c. with a full glass of water

d. at bedtime

10. Your client has a feeding tube. You receive the following order: Administer full strength Isocal (240 mL can), 2000 mL daily. At what rate will you set the infusion pump?

a. 50 mL/hr

b. 83 mL/hr

c. 93 mL/hr

d. 250 mL/hr

CHAPTER 27

Drugs for Weight Management

■ Exercises

Match the following.

1. _____lipokinetix

2. _____glucomannan

3. _____sibutramine (Meridia)

4. _____hydroxycitric acid

5. _____orlistat (Xenical)

6. _____fenfluramine

7. _____guar gum

8. _____ephedra

9. _____phentermine (Ionamin)

10. _____St. John's wort

a. Thought to produce weight loss by increasing serotonin and norepinephrine

b. May increase blood pressure and heart rate

c. Pharmacologically and chemically similar to amphetamines

d. A weight loss drug taken off the market in 1997

e. Decreases absorption of dietary fat from the intestine

f. Produces feelings of stomach fullness, causing a person to eat less

g. Dietary fiber that is bulk forming and found in weight-loss products

h. Associated with severe hepatotoxicity

i. An herb used in many weight-loss products

j. Suppresses appetite in animals

Place T (true) or F (false) in each blank.

1. _____ Obesity is considered a major health problem.

2. _____ Obesity is more likely to occur in poor people.

3. _____ Treatment for obesity is recommended for people who have a BMI of 20 kg/m2.

4. _____ Use of amphetamines for weight control is encouraged.

5. _____ Ephedra-containing products contain caffeine.

6. _____ Guarana is safe to use in peptic ulcer disease.

7. _____ A multivitamin containing fat-soluble vitamins should be taken two hours before administration of orlistat (Xenical).

8. _____ When drug therapy is indicated for obesity, a single drug in the lowest effective dose is recommended.

9. _____ A client taking an appetite suppressant who has not lost four pounds during the first month of treatment will probably not lose weight with the drug.

10. _____ The recommended rate of weight loss is approximately five pounds a week.

■ Clinical Challenge

A mother brings her 10-year-old son to the clinic. She tells you that she wants the doctor to prescribe a medicine that will help her son lose weight. She says he eats all the time. Assessment reveals that he is 4 feet 8 inches and weighs 180 pounds. The mother works 10 hours a day and the son stays with his 87-year-old grandfather when he is not in school. How do you respond?

Outline a teaching plan for the mother and her son.

■ Review Questions

1. Phentermine (Ionamin), an adrenergic anorexiant, has been prescribed for your client. Which of the following conditions is a contraindication to the use of this drug?
   a. diabetes mellitus
   b. cardiovascular disease
   c. chronic fatigue syndrome
   d. confusion

2. Which of the following statements by your client leads you to believe that she has a good under-standing of the drug orlistat (Xenical)?
   a. "I hate having to take the medication three times a day."
   b. "I no longer have a lot of gas."
   c. "I take a multivitamin with my morning dose of Xenical."
   d. "I shouldn't have as many bowel movements as I have been having."

3. You are working with an obese client who tells you that she does not like to leave her house, even to go to the grocery store. She states that she has had her groceries delivered to her home for the past 2 years. Which of the following would be an appropriate nursing diagnosis for her?
   a. imbalanced nutrition, more than body requirements
   b. activity intolerance related to weight
   c. chronic low self-esteem related to body image
   d. fluid volume excess related to excessive intake

4. Amphetamines are not recommended for weight management because of their:
   a. serious adverse effects
   b. high potential for abuse and dependence
   c. cost to the client
   d. action to increase energy level and decrease gastric secretion

5. Your client asks you how sibutramine (Meridia) will help him lose weight. Your response would be:
   a. "This drug will decrease your appetite and cause a faster metabolism rate."
   b. "It will increase your energy level and decrease gastric secretions."
   c. "It produces a feeling of fullness and causes esophageal irritation."
   d. "It decreases absorption of dietary fat from the intestines."

6. Your client is taking orlistat (Xenical) for weight management. To avoid abdominal cramping and gas pains sometimes associated with this drug you would instruct her to:
   a. drink eight glasses of water a day
   b. avoid large amounts of fatty foods
   c. take an antispasmodic when symptoms occur
   d. eliminate caffeine from her diet

7. You are instructing your client on the use of sibu-tramine (Meridia). Instructions will include to:
   a. take one capsule with each main meal or up to three capsules a day
   b. take two pills at night before going to bed
   c. take one dose daily in the morning with or without food
   d. take a single dose mid-morning

8. A client has a BMI of 27.5 kg/m². The value would indicate that the client is:

a. underweight

b. within normal weight range

c. overweight

d. obese

9. A client of Asian descent comes to the weight management clinic for help. Which of the following drugs will *not* be prescribed for this client?

a. diethylpropion (Tenuate)

b. sibutramine (Meridia)

c. phendimetrazine (Bontril)

d. Lipokinetix

10. A common side effect of phentermine (Ionamin) is:

a. dry mouth

b. diarrhea

c. hypotension

d. lethargy

CHAPTER 28

General Characteristics of Antimicrobial Drugs

■ Exercises

Match the following.

1. ____ anaerobic bacteria

2. ____ viruses

3. ____ *Escherichia coli*

4. ____ nosocomial infection

5. ____ streptococci

6. ____ aerobic bacteria

7. ____ pathogenic

8. ____ "opportunistic" microorganism

9. ____ bactericidal

10. ____ fungi

a. Intracellular parasites that survive only in living tissue

b. Bacteria that require oxygen

c. Normal endogenous or environmental flora

d. An infection acquired in a hospital

e. Plant-like organisms that live as parasites on living tissue

f. A drug that kills a microorganism

g. Part of normal microbial flora of throat and nasopharynx

h. Disease-producing

i. An organism that most often causes urinary tract infections

j. Bacteria that cannot live in the presence of oxygen

Complete the chart by placing a check mark in the appropriate column.

Bacteria pathogen	Gram-positive; gram-negative	Normal body flora	Medical conditions
E. coli			
Enterococci			
Staphylococcus spp.			
Bacteroides spp.			
Klebsiella spp.			
Streptococcus spp.			

Answer the following.

1. List the major defense mechanisms of the body.

2. List contributing factors for the increasing prevalence of antibiotic-resistant microorganisms.

3. List the mechanisms of action for antimicrobial drugs.

■ Review Questions

1. It is important to administer antimicrobial drugs at scheduled, evenly spaced intervals to ensure:
   a. use of all packaged medication
   b. therapeutic blood levels
   c. minimal adverse effects
   d. client compliance

2. Which of the following outcomes would be appropriate for a client receiving antimicrobial therapy who has a wound infection?
   a. decrease in white blood cell count
   b. increase in malaise and lethargy
   c. increase in drainage
   d. decrease in appetite

3. Most intravenous administration of antimicrobial drugs should infuse over:
   a. 5 to 10 minutes
   b. 15 to 30 minutes
   c. 30 to 60 minutes
   d. 60 to 90 minutes

4. Which of the following adverse effects will occur with most antimicrobial agents?
   a. diarrhea
   b. nausea
   c. headache
   d. hypersensitivity

5. You have an order to mix an antibiotic with multivitamins in 50 cc of solution and administer intravenously over 1 hour. Which of the following nursing measures is most appropriate?
   a. Prepare and administer the order as written.
   b. Check with the head nurse before administration of the IV medications.
   c. Call the physician to clarify the order.

   d. Decrease the amount of solution used to mix the antibiotic powder because the multivitamins will be added to the antibiotics.

6. A client has been receiving antimicrobial therapy for 2 weeks. He has lost 7 pounds during that time. When the nurse questions him concerning the weight loss, he tells her he doesn't feel like eating. The most appropriate nursing diagnosis for this client would be:
   a. fatigue related to infection
   b. deficient knowledge: use of antimicrobial drugs
   c. imbalanced nutrition: less than body requirements related to adverse effects of drug therapy
   d. risk for injury: related to adverse drug effects

7. The most effective method of preventing infection is:
   a. accurate administration of antibiotics
   b. the use of isolation procedures
   c. keeping skin clean and dry
   d. handwashing

8. If severe adverse effects of antimicrobial therapy occur, clients should:
   a. stop the drug immediately
   b. continue taking the medication until it is all gone
   c. report adverse effects to health care provider immediately
   d. decrease the dosage and continue therapy

9. Which of the following laboratory tests identifies infectious agents by measuring the titer in the serum of a diseased host?
   a. Gram's stain
   b. culture
   c. serology
   d. detection of antigens

10. The duration for antimicrobial therapy is usually:
   a. 3 to 5 days
   b. 7 to 10 days
   c. 12 to 15 days
   d. 14 to 21 days

CHAPTER 29

Beta-Lactam Antibacterials: Penicillins, Cephalosporins, and Others

■ Exercises

Answer the following.

1. List four groups of beta-lactam antibiotics.

2. Describe the mechanism of action for beta-lactam antibacterial drugs.

3. Explain how a beta-lactamase inhibitor, when combined with a penicillin, produces a therapeutic effect.

4. Why might some clients be allergic to both penicillins and cephalosporins?

Match the following.

1. ____ amoxicillin (Amoxil)

2. ____ nafcillin (Unipen)

3. ____ cephalosporins

4. ____ cefoxitin (Mefoxin)

5. ____ penicillin G

6. ____ aztreonam (Azactam)

7. ____ ampicillin

8. ____ imipenem/cilastatin (Primaxin)

9. ____ penicillin V

10. ____ carbenicillin

a. An extended-spectrum/antipseudomonal penicillin used to treat urinary tract infections and prostatitis

b. Active against *Bacteroides fragilis*, an anaerobic organism resistant to most drugs

c. Administered only by the oral route

d. A monobactam active against gram-negative bacteria

e. A broad-spectrum, semisynthetic penicillin used for gram-negative and gram-positive bacterial infections

f. A carbapenem that requires lidocaine to be added for an IM injection to decrease pain

g. Penicillinase-resistant penicillin

h. Broad-spectrum antibacterial agents that come from fungus

i. Prototype for penicillins

j. An aminopenicillin that is converted to ampicillin in the body

Place T (true) or F (false) in each blank.

1. ____ Beta-lactam antibiotics are most effective when bacterial cells are dividing.

2. ____ The most serious adverse effect of the penicillins is nephropathy.

3. ____ Penicillins are more effective in infections caused by gram-negative bacteria.

4. ____ An allergic reaction to one penicillin usually means a client will be allergic to all penicillins.

5. ____ In general, cephalosporins are more active against gram-positive organisms.

6. ____ Third-generation cephalosporins are used to treat meningeal infections.

7. ____ Penicillins are more effective in most streptococcal and staphylococcal infections.

8. ____ Penicillin is the most common cause of drug-induced anaphylaxis.

9. ____ Second-generation cephalosporins are often used for surgical prophylaxis with prosthetic implants.

10. ____ In the hospital setting, the intramuscular route is always used for the administration of penicillin.

■ Clinical Challenge

Your client is an 11-year-old male who has a positive throat culture for streptococci. He is given a prescription for amoxicillin capsules 250 mg every 8 hours PO for 10 days. What should your teaching plan include? What should you tell the client and his mother about taking the medication at school?

■ Review Questions

1. A 28-year-old female has been given a prescription for cefdinir (Omnicef) 300 mg every 12 hours for bronchitis. Which of the following statements by her indicates that she has an understanding of cefdinir therapy?

   a. "I take my medication on an empty stomach."

   b. "I take my medication every 4 hours."

   c. "I take my antibiotic right before breakfast and before my evening meal."

   d. "I will take this medication as long as my throat hurts."

2. A client is 73 years old and is taking a cephalosporin. There is a possibility that this client may develop:

   a. nephrotoxicity

   b. pernicious anemia

   c. fibromyalgia

   d. endocarditis

3. When explaining to your client that he should not drink cranberry or orange juice while taking Nafcillin, you will advise him that:

   a. if acidic juices are ingested, solid foods should be taken with penicillin

   b. oral penicillins are destroyed by acids

   c. acids increase the absorption rate of penicillins

   d. acids increase the blood level of penicillins

4. Imipenem (Primaxin) is contraindicated in clients with:

   a. anemia

   b. hypertension

   c. diabetes mellitus

   d. seizure disorders

5. A client is to begin Penicillin V therapy. The nurse is aware that this drug is to be administered:

   a. orally

   b. subcutaneously

   c. intramuscularly

   d. intravenously

6. Which of the following electrolyte imbalances may occur with the use of large doses of IV penicillin G potassium?

   a. hypokalemia

   b. hyperkalemia

   c. hyponatremia

   d. hypernatremia

7. Your client has cancer of both kidneys. Which of the following will be important in determining the correct dosage of a cephalosporin?

   a. urinary output

   b. creatinine clearance level

   c. 24-hour urine

   d. urine pH

8. When teaching a young mother about administration of a penicillin, the home care nurse will advise:

   a. shaking the liquid suspension to resuspend the medication before giving it

   b. warming the medication prior to administration

   c. administering with a fruit juice

   d. giving only when the child is awake

9. You are the medication nurse for an 8-hour shift. You must give ampicillin IM. In planning for preparation of all the medications on the floor that you will be giving, you are aware that reconstituted ampicillin must be given:

   a. with breakfast

   b. within 15 minutes of preparation

   c. in the deltoid muscle

   d. within 1 hour of preparation

10. Your client is taking a cephalosporin for a urinary tract infection. Which of the following drugs would you inform your client that he should not take with the cephalosporin therapy?

   a. Lanoxin

   b. Mylanta

   c. erythromycin

   d. Valium

CHAPTER 30

Aminoglycosides, Fluoroquinolones, Macrolides, and Miscellaneous Antibacterials

■ Exercises

Match the following.

1. _____ azithromycin

2. _____ chloramphenicol (chloromycetin)

3. _____ Linezolid (Zyrox)

4. _____ gentamicin

5. _____ spectinomycin (Trobicin)

6. _____ telithromycin (Ketek)

7. _____ clindamycin (Cleocin)

8. _____ quinupristin/dalfopristin (Synercid)

9. _____ erythromycin

10. _____ clarithromycin

a. Used to treat *Helicobacter pylori* infections associated with peptic ulcer disease

b. Myelosuppression may result from use

c. Prototype for macrolides

d. Indicated for skin and skin structure infections

e. Used to treat urethritis and cervicitis

f. Used to treat gonococcal infections

g. Aminoglycoside prototype

h. Used to treat infections caused by *B. fragilis* and gram-negative organisms from the gynecologic or gastrointestinal tracts

i. New drug used in the treatment of *Streptococcus pneumoniae*

j. Used to treat serous infections for which no adequate substitute drug is available

Place T (true) or F (false) in each blank.

1. _____ Aminoglycosides are used to treat serious gram-positive infections.

2. _____ Many nosocomial infections are caused by gram-negative organism.

3. _____ Smaller doses of aminoglycosides are indicated for urinary tract infections.

4. _____ Fluoroquinolones are synthetic bactericidal drugs used to treat gram-negative and gram-positive organisms.

5. _____ Children younger than 12 years of age should not take fluoroquinolones.

6. _____ Azithromycin increases carbamazepine levels.

7. _____ Macrolides are contraindicated in people who have preexisting liver disease.

8. _____ Most oral erythromycin should be taken with food.

9. _____ Neomycin is not recommended for use in infants and children.

10. _____ Vancomycin is indicated only for the treatment of severe infections.

■ Clinical Challenge

Your client is being treated with ciprofloxacin (Cipro) for gonorrhea. What assessment data are needed before therapy is started? What instructions will you give to the client?

Your client is a 52-year-old female who has peritonitis. She has been taking clindamycin hydrochloride (Cleocin) 300 mg PO every 6 hours for 5 days. She reports fever and severe diarrhea with pus and blood. What do you suspect? What do you tell her?

She asks you how she got these infections when she was already taking an antibiotic. How do you respond? What will be her treatment plan?

■ Review Questions

1. Your client is to start on tobramycin (Nebcin) for a nosocomial infection. Which of the following would be the most helpful in determining the correct dosage of Nebcin?

   a. the client's blood pressure

   b. the client's weight

   c. what time the client eats breakfast

   d. other client medication

2. Clients who are on aminoglycoside therapy would be assessed for factors that could predispose to:

   a. cardiotoxicity and hepatotoxicity

   b. diabetes mellitus and nephrotoxicity

   c. ototoxicity and hypertension

   d. nephrotoxicity and ototoxicity

3. Your client is to receive clindamycin (Cleocin). In order to promote therapeutic effects, you will administer the drug:

   a. with a fruit juice

   b. with a light snack

   c. when the client has an empty stomach

   d. with meals

4. Linezolid (Zyvox) is being given to your client for pneumonia. You will stress:

   a. weekly CBC monitoring

   b. daily weights

   c. increase in caloric intake

   d. blood pressure monitoring

5. Gentamicin (Garamycin) is begun for your client. Which laboratory value should be monitored?

   a. potassium level

   b. serum creatinine level

   c. serum albumin level

   d. prothrombin time

6. Erythromycin can interfere with the elimination of other drugs. Which of the following explains why toxicity of the other drugs may occur?

   a. The affected drugs are eliminated more slowly, increasing their serum levels.

   b. The affected drugs are eliminated very quickly, decreasing their serum levels.

   c. Erythromycin causes an increase in metabolism of the other drugs.

   d. Erythromycin can cause an antagonistic effect when given with other drugs.

7. Your client is taking gentamicin. A trough level should be obtained:

   a. 15 to 30 minutes before the next dose

   b. 1 hour before the next dose

   c. 2 hours before the next dose

   d. 30 minutes after the next dose

8. Your client has *Haemophilus* meningitis. He is allergic to penicillin and has been placed on chloramphenicol. He should be closely monitored for:

   a. diabetes mellitus

   b. blood dyscrasia

   c. hepatic toxicity

   d. ototoxicity

9. Your client has a severe systemic infection and is being treated with vancomycin IV. You will monitor the client for:

   a. decrease in blood pressure and flushing

   b. increase in fever and heart rate

   c. shortness of breath and dizziness

   d. increase in blood pressure and itching

10. Your client has been taking ciprofloxacin (Cipro) for 3 days for pneumonia. She calls the clinic and reports that she has an itchy rash all over her body. You advise her to:

    a. stop taking the drug immediately

    b. request a topical cream for the rash

    c. decrease the dosage of Cipro

    d. continue the drug as ordered

CHAPTER 31

Tetracyclines, Sulfonamides, and Urinary Agents

■ Exercises

Answer the following.

1. List four clinical indications for tetracyclines.

2. Describe the mechanism of action for tetracyclines.

3. Describe the mechanism of action for sulfonamides.

4. Why are tetracyclines contraindicated in pregnant women and children up to 8 years of age?

Place T (true) or F (false) in each blank.

1. ____ Tetracyclines may be substituted for penicillin in treating streptococcal pharyngitis.

2. ____ Tetracyclines should not be substituted for penicillin in serious staphylococcal infections.

3. ____ Sulfasalazine (Azulfidine) is contraindicated in people who are allergic to salicylates.

4. ____ Urinary antiseptics can be used to treat urinary tract infections and ulcerative colitis.

5. ____ Doxycycline can be used in clients with renal failure.

6. ____ The intramuscular route is preferred for tetracycline therapy.

7. ____ With sulfonamide therapy, alkaline urine decreases drug solubility.

8. ____ Urine pH must be acidic for Mandelamine therapy to be therapeutic.

9. ____ Sulfonamides may be used to treat urinary tract infections in children older than 2 months.

10. ____ With the combination of sulfamethoxazole (Bactrim) and trimethoprim (Septra), older adults are at risk for bone marrow depression.

▪ Clinical Challenge

A client comes to the clinic complaining of signs and symptoms of a urinary tract infection. After a thorough assessment, you determine that the client is allergic to penicillin and "sulfur" drugs. The nurse indicates the allergies on the client's chart. A urinalysis does indicate that the client has a urinary tract infection. The physician orders sulfamethoxazole and trimethoprim (Septra). What should the nurse do?

▪ Review Questions

1. Your client, age 19, has been on tetracycline therapy for 3 years. Which of the following should be monitored?
   a. blood pressure
   b. liver function
   c. blood glucose level
   d. renal function

2. When instructing a client who will be taking tetracycline for the first time the nurse should include which of the following?
   a. Take medication with glass of milk.
   b. It is permissible to take an antacid within 30 minutes of taking medication.
   c. Out-of-date medication may be used.
   d. Keep container of medication in a cabinet away from light.

3. Which of the following statements by your client indicates that she does not have an understanding of doxycycline (Vibramycin) therapy?
   a. "I will be spending my summer at the beach."
   b. "I will take my medication by mouth."
   c. "If I experience perineal itching, I will let my doctor know."
   d. "I take my medication with saltine crackers."

4. When instructing a client concerning tetracycline therapy, which of the following should be included in your teaching plan?
   a. The intramuscular route is preferred.
   b. Avoid dairy product ingestion with tetracycline.
   c. Outdated tetracycline may be used up to 1 year.
   d. Always take all tetracycline on an empty stomach.

5. Which of the following drugs is used as prophylaxis for recurrent urinary tract infections?
   a. nitrofurantoin (Macrodantin)
   b. trimethoprim (Trimpex)
   c. fosfomycin (Monurol)
   d. mafenide (Sulfamylon)

6. A 30-year-old female comes to the clinic complaining of dysuria, burning, and frequency and urgency of urination. A urinalysis indicates she has a urinary tract infection. The physician prescribes sulfamethoxazole (Gantanol). Which of the following drugs may also be prescribed to relieve her discomfort?
   a. methenamine mandelate (Mandelamine)
   b. phenazopyridine (Pyridium)
   c. fosfomycin (Monurol)
   d. sulfamethizole (Thiosulfil)

7. Your client is being treated for Rocky Mountain Spotted fever. He is taking tetracycline (Achromycin) 2 gm/day in 4 equal doses. He complains of soreness and white patches in his mouth, and states that his tongue has turned black. You suspect that:
   a. his condition has worsened
   b. he has a monilial superinfection
   c. he is having adverse effects from the Achromycin
   d. he is having an allergic reaction to a food substance

8. Your client will be taking sulfamethoxazole, trimethoprim (Bactrim) for an extended period of time. Which of the following laboratory tests would *not* be included in periodic clinic visits?

   a. aspartate aminotransferase levels

   b. blood urea nitrogen

   c. pulmonary function

   d. hematuria

9. A client is to be placed on sulfasalazine (Azulfidine) for ulcerative colitis. Which of the following drugs being taken by the client should be reported to his physician?

   a. Fosamax

   b. aspirin

   c. Synthroid

   d. Inderal

10. The client is taking fosfomycin (Monurol) for a urinary tract infection. The nurse is aware that administration of this drug is:

    a. without food

    b. with a full glass of water

    c. immediately after the powder is mixed with water

    d. three times a day

CHAPTER 32

Drugs for Tuberculosis and *Mycobacterium avium* Complex (MAC) Disease

■ Exercises

Answer the following.

1. Describe the physiological action of isoniazid (INH).

2. Differentiate latent tuberculosis infection (LTBI) from active tuberculosis (TB).

3. What is a major concern among public health care providers concerning tuberculosis?

4. How can nurses help control the spread of TB?

5. Name five primary drugs used to treat TB.

Match the following.

1. _____ rifampin (Rifadin)

2. _____ pyrazinamide

3. _____ capreomycin (Capastat)

4. _____ isoniazid (INH)

5. _____ ofloxacin

6. _____ streptomycin

7. _____ rifabutin (Mycobutin)

8. _____ ethambutol (Myambutol)

9. _____ rifapentine (Priftin)

10. _____ azithromycin

a. Used to treat pulmonary tuberculosis; less frequent administration than rifampin

b. An antitubercular drug that inhibits synthesis of ribonucleic acid and interferes with mycobacterial protein metabolism

c. Synergistic in combination with isoniazid (INH) to kill tuberculosis bacilli

d. Used with INH and rifampin for the first 2 months of active tuberculosis treatment

e. Used in the prevention of MAC disease

f. A fluoroquinolone that can be used to treat multidrug-resistant tuberculosis in adults

g. Most commonly used antitubercular drug

h. Indicated for use only when other drugs used for tuberculosis are contraindicated

i. An aminoglycoside antibiotic used in a medication regimen for tuberculosis

j. Used in clients with HIV who have *Mycobacterium avium* complex and as a substitute for rifampin.

Place T (true) or F (false) in each blank.

1. ____ Multidrug-resistant tuberculosis (MDR-TB) indicates organisms that are resistant to isoniazid (INH) and rifampin.

2. ____ A major change in the treatment of tuberculosis is increasing use of short-course regimens.

3. ____ Pyrazinamide is contraindicated during pregnancy.

4. ____ INH therapy should be once a week.

5. ____ Screening for tuberculosis is done only at public health departments.

6. ____ Prophylactic drug therapy for *mycobacterium avium* and *mycobacterium intracellulare* is lifelong.

7. ____ Hepatitis is more likely to occur during the first 8 weeks of INH therapy.

8. ____ INH therapy is questioned in older adults, due to the increased risk of drug-induced hepatotoxicity.

9. ____ Rifampin increases blood levels and therapeutic effects of anti-HIV drugs.

10. ____ INH increases blood levels of phenytoin (Dilantin).

■ Clinical Challenge

You are a home health nurse, and you are planning a visit to a 78-year-old Hispanic female who lives with her daughter and son-in-law, and their four children. Your client has active TB and has just returned home after 2 weeks in the hospital. What do you plan for your first home visit?

■ Review Questions

1. Your client, age 43, has been diagnosed with active tuberculosis. He is taking multiple drug therapy, including INH and rifampin (Rifadin). Which of the following laboratory tests should be done at least once a month?

   a. serum alanine, aspartate aminotransferases (ALT and AST), and bilirubin

   b. red blood count, white blood count, and differential

   c. thyroid-stimulating hormone, thyroxine, and triiodothyronine levels

   d. fasting blood sugar and 2-hour postprandial blood sugar

2. INH therapy has been started on your client. You have completed a thorough assessment. Of the following prescribed drugs for the client, which one should be reported to the client's physician?

   a. acetaminophen (Tylenol)

   b. vitamin B_6

   c. diltiazem hydrochloride (Cardizem)

   d. folic acid

3. When teaching clients concerning the use of antituberculosis drugs, a nurse would advise which of the following?

   a. There is no need for concern of liver damage.

   b. Drug therapy for tuberculosis is a lifetime commitment.

   c. Drug therapy lasts only a couple of months.

   d. Hypersensitivity reactions are more likely to occur between the third and eighth week of drug therapy.

4. A 28-year-old female is being treated for active TB with INH and rifampin (Rifadin). She should be informed that:

   a. she should have her blood glucose levels checked at least every month while on drug therapy

   b. she should use additional birth control if she is taking an oral contraceptive

   c. she will probably gain weight while on TB drug therapy

   d. she will most likely have to take the medication for 2 to 3 years

5. Your client who has active TB asks you how long it will take the medication to make him feel better. An appropriate response would be:

    a. "Don't worry about that. You are going to feel better soon."

    b. "You will probably be on the medication for about a year."

    c. "You should begin to feel better within 2 to 3 weeks of starting the medications."

    d. "That's really hard to predict."

6. Which of the following groups of people who may be on INH therapy are more likely to have serious liver impairment?

    a. Asians

    b. alcoholics

    c. diabetics

    d. homeless

7. Why should rifampin therapy not be used in people with HIV?

    a. Rifampin increases the severity of the anti-HIV drugs' adverse effects.

    b. Rifampin increases blood levels and therapeutic effects of anti-HIV drugs.

    c. Rifampin's therapeutic effects are decreased by the anti-HIV drugs.

    d. Rifampin decreases blood levels and therapeutic effects of anti-HIV drugs.

8. Your client has recently been diagnosed with active TB and is taking INH and rifampin. Pyrazinamide is also added for the first 2 months of therapy. Which of the following laboratory tests should be done during the first 2 months of therapy in relation to pyrazinamide?

    a. blood urea nitrogen levels

    b. uric acid levels

    c. creatinine levels

    d. urine osmolality

9. A client is receiving ethambutol as part of a four-drug regimen for TB. Which of the following may be of concern for this client?

    a. driving his car in town

    b. eating a high protein, low-fat diet

    c. playing tennis every weekend

    d. smoking a pack of cigarettes per day

10. Your client is taking rifampin (Rifadin) for active TB. When discussing this drug with the client, you should stress that:

    a. the drug does not cause gastrointestinal upset

    b. the drug can cause seizures

    c. a "butterfly rash" may appear across the face but will go away once therapy is concluded

    d. the red/orange discoloration of urine is a side effect but is harmless

CHAPTER 33

Antiviral, Antifungal, and Antiparasitic Drugs

Match the following.

1. ____ *candida albicans*

2. ____ ritonavir

3. ____ oseltamivir (Tamiflu)

4. ____ fluconazole (Diflucan)

5. ____ acyclovir

6. ____ terbinafine (Lamisil)

7. ____ giardiasis

8. ____ viruses

9. ____ nystatin (Mycostatin)

10. ____ griseofulvin (Fulvicin)

11. ____ zidovudine (AZT)

12. ____ amphotericin B (Fungizone)

13. ____ toxoplasmosis

14. ____ fungi

15. ____ chloroquine (Aralen)

16. ____ metronidazole (Flagyl)

17. ____ itraconazole (Sporanox)

18. ____ famciclovir

19. ____ amantadine

20. ____ parasites

a. Prototype for Nucleoside Reverse Transcriptase Inhibitors

b. Drug of choice for histoplasmosis

c. Normal microbial flora of the skin, mouth, GI tract, and vagina

d. Can treat vaginal candidiasis in a single oral dose

e. Antifungal drug that should be taken with fatty foods

f. A living organism that survives at the expense of another organism

g. Oral drug used to treat fungal infection of nails

h. Caused by an intestinal parasite and can be found in people who camp or hike in wilderness areas.

i. Intracellular parasites that can live and reproduce while inside other cells

j. An agent used topically to treat oral, intestinal, or vaginal candidiasis

k. Used to treat herpes zoster

l. Used to treat influenza A infections

m. Increases sedation and respiratory depression when used with benzodiazepines

n. Caused by ingesting undercooked meat or contact with feces from infected cats

o. Used to treat malaria

p. Molds and yeasts found in the environment

q. Used to treat influenza A or B

r. Systemic treatment for trichomoniasis

s. Antifungal drug used to treat serious systemic fungal infections

t. Used in the treatment of genital herpes

Place T (true) or F (false) in each blank.

1. _____ Drug therapy for viral infections is limited.

2. _____ Most antiviral agents eliminate viruses from tissues.

3. _____ Live attenuated viral vaccines may be used in women who are pregnant.

4. _____ Dosage of acyclovir must be reduced in the presence of renal impairment.

5. _____ Most invasive fungal infections are acquired by inhalation of airborne spores.

6. _____ Systemic fungal infections are decreasing in incidence.

7. _____ Nephrotoxicity is the most common and most serious long term adverse effect of amphotericin B.

8. _____ All azoles are contraindicated during pregnancy.

9. _____ Amebiasis is a common disease found in the United States.

10. _____ Primaquine can be used to prevent the recurrence of malaria.

Complete the chart.

Drug	Parasitic Infection
mebendazole (Vermox)	
pyrantel (Antiminth)	
thiabendazole (Mintezol)	
permethrin (Elimite)	
malathion (Ovide)	

■ Clinical Challenge

Your client is a 23-year-old female who has just been diagnosed with HIV. She is to start on zidovudine and ritonavir. She is extremely upset and keeps saying she cannot believe this is happening to her. How do you approach her concerning drug therapy? What specific instructions do you give her concerning these drugs?

Your client is a 72-year-old male who has battled emphysema for many years. He is admitted to the hospital with a possible diagnosis of aspergillosis. He is started on amphotericin B. Which adverse effects will you look for? If the client develops hypertension, edema, or hypokalemia, what should you do?

A client is going on a medical/construction mission trip to Africa. She is in the clinic for her physical exam and immunization update. The nurse discusses the need for malaria prophylaxis. The physician prescribes chloroquine with primaquine. What will the nurse teach the client regarding these drugs?

■ Review Questions

1. Your client is a 42-year-old male who was recently diagnosed with AIDS. He is to begin drug therapy with zidovudine (AZT) 300 mg PO. You will anticipate which of the following dosage schedules?

    a. every 4 hours

    b. twice a day

    c. three times a day

    d. four times a day

2. Before clients are placed on amprenavir (Agenerase), they should be assessed for an allergic reaction to which of the following drugs?

    a. penicillins

    b. sulfonamides

    c. benzodiazepines

    d. acetaminophens

3. Your client has been diagnosed with influenza A, and amantadine (Symmetrel) has been prescribed for her. You will inform her of which of the following side effects?

   a. insomnia

   b. headache

   c. palpitations

   d. burning sensation in hands and feet

4. Which of the following drugs is given for prevention of influenza in children?

   a. amantadine (Symmetrel)

   b. zanamivir (Relenza)

   c. oseltamivir (Tamiflu)

   d. rimantadine (Flumadine)

5. Your client has tinea pedis. Haloprogin (Halotex) 1% cream daily has been prescribed. Which of the following instructions should be given to the client?

   a. Wash hair before applying cream to scalp.

   b. Wash and dry feet before applying the cream.

   c. Do not wet area before application of cream.

   d. Apply cream and remove after 30 minutes.

6. Which of the following is the most common and most serious adverse effect of amphotericin B?

   a. hepatoxicity

   b. cardiotoxicity

   c. nephrotoxicity

   d. ototoxicity

7. Your client has a diagnosis of oral *candidiasis*. Which of the following drugs do you expect her to be placed on?

   a. nystatin (Mycostatin)

   b. natamycin (Natacyn)

   c. naftifine (Naftin)

   d. ketoconazole (Nizoral)

8. When teaching a young mother about treatment of pediculosis capitis for her 5-year-old, the nurse will stress the importance of:

   a. drug therapy, including measures to avoid reinfection or transmission to others

   b. keeping her child from playing in the dirt

   c. keeping the child isolated from other children for at least 2 weeks

   d. Avoiding raw fish and undercooked meat

9. You are taking care of a missionary who has spent a year in Asia. He is being treated with iodoquinol (Yodoxin) for intestinal amebiasis. Which of the following statement would you expect from your client?

   a. "I'm not sure where I am."

   b. "I'm experiencing severe headaches."

   c. "I have heartburn."

   d. "I wish this nausea would go away."

10. When instructing a client who has malaria regarding administration of chloroquine (Aralen), the nurse should include:

    a. Take medication with or after meals.

    b. Drink a full glass of water with each dose.

    c. Take 2 hours before meals.

    d. Avoid dairy products when taking the medication.

CHAPTER 34

Immunizing Agents

■ Exercises

Place a T (true) or F (false) in each blank.

1. ____ Antigens that activate the immune response can be microorganisms that cause infectious diseases.

2. ____ It is recommended that only activated polio vaccine be used in the United States.

3. ____ Hepatitis B virus (HBV) infection can cause liver disease.

4. ____ HBV is recommended for at-risk people only.

5. ____ Immunization against diphtheria and tetanus is one time only for life.

6. ____ Vaccines should *not* be given together.

7. ____ Immunization involves administration of an antibody to produce an antigen.

8. ____ Attenuated vaccines are weakened or reduced in virulence, which can cause mild forms of the disease.

9. ____ Most often, attenuated live vaccines produce lifelong immunity.

10. ____ Toxoids are chemical toxins that have been changed to destroy toxicity yet still are able to initiate antibody formation.

11. ____ Toxoid immunity is *not* permanent, and repeated doses are needed.

12. ____ Vaccines containing aluminum should be given by mouth.

13. ____ Vaccines and toxoids should not be given during febrile illnesses.

14. ____ The best source for information concerning current recommendations is the Centers for Disease Control and Prevention (CDC).

15. ____ The measles-mumps-rubella (MMR) vaccine should be stored away from light.

16. ____ Most vaccines require refrigeration.

17. ____ MMR is given to infants at 6 months of age.

18. ____ Pneumococcal vaccine is *not* recommended for children.

19. ____ Varicella vaccine should be given twice by 12 years of age.

20. ____ Health care workers should have a tetanus-diphtheria booster every 10 years.

21. ____ High-risk groups and health care providers should receive the influenza vaccine annually.

22. ____ Adults born before 1957 are considered immune to measles.

23. ____ Live vaccines should *not* be given to people with cancer.

24. ____ Children with HIV infection should receive all immunizations.

25. ____ *Haemophilus influenzae* type b (Hib) conjugate vaccine is given to prevent serious bacterial infections, including meningitis.

■ Clinical Challenge

A mother of a pre-college student calls the clinic and is clearly upset. She explains that her son is being denied admission to the college of his choice because he does not have an immunization record. After asking her a few questions, you determine that her husband is in the military and that they have lived in seven states over the past 15 years. She tells you that she is sure that her son received all vaccines, but she can't find the immunization card. What do you tell her? What would you tell a new mother concerning recordkeeping of immunizations?

■ Review Questions

1. A mother has brought her 15-month-old daughter to the health department for diphtheria-tetanus-pertussis (DTaP) and MMR vaccines. Which of the following drugs should be suggested for fever and soreness at the injection site?
   a. Aspirin
   b. Advil
   c. Tylenol
   d. Motrin

2. A 20-year-old female is given a rubella immunization. Which of the following statements by the nurse is *most* important?
   a. "You may take Tylenol for the fever and pain."
   b. "You must use effective birth control for at least 3 months."
   c. "You may experience flu-like symptoms."
   d. "You should take it easy for about 3 days."

3. A young mother has brought her 6-month-old baby into the clinic for immunizations. The nurse should assess for:
   a. fever
   b. weight loss
   c. anemia
   d. slowed development

4. After a baby receives a DTaP the nurse will teach the mother to watch for which of the following potential adverse effects?
   a. anorexia and nausea
   b. tremors and possible seizures
   c. difficulty swallowing and abdominal distention
   d. diarrhea and abdominal pain

5. Which of the following drugs decrease the overall effects of vaccines?
   a. acetaminophen (Tylenol)
   b. diazepam (Valium)
   c. furosemide (Lasix)
   d. phenytoin (Dilantin)

6. In assessing immunization needs of your client who will be leaving for Asia in several weeks, you explain that he should receive a tetanus toxoid injection if he has not had one in the last:
   a. 6 months
   b. year
   c. 5 years
   d. 10 years

7. The hepatitis B vaccine is recommended as early as:
   a. within 12 hours of birth
   b. 6 months of age
   c. 1 year of age
   d. 6 years of age

8. You must give RhoGAM to your Rh-negative client who just delivered an Rh-positive baby within:
   a. 1 hour
   b. 6 hours
   c. 24 hours
   d. 72 hours

9. You have just administered vaccines to three children. You explained to their mother that she must wait with the children in the clinic for at least:
    a. 15 minutes
    b. 30 minutes
    c. 1 hour
    d. 1½ hours

10. Which of the following drugs should be readily available when administering any immunization?
    a. Tylenol
    b. Valium
    c. Epinephrine
    d. Lasix

CHAPTER 35

Hematopoietic and Immunostimulant Drugs

■ Exercises

Answer the following.

1. Why are hematopoietic and immunostimulant drugs given?

2. What are the disadvantages of using cytokines?

3. How do interferons weaken viruses?

4. How does bacillus Calmette-Guérin (BCG) vaccine act against cancer of the urinary bladder?

5. Why are hematopoietic and immunostimulant drugs given subcutaneously or intravenously?

Fill in the blank.

1. _____ is used to prevent severe thrombocytopenia and reduces the need for platelet transfusions in clients with cancer who are taking chemotherapy.

2. _____ are used to treat viral infections and cancers.

3. _____ _____ and _____ are used to treat or prevent anemia.

4. _____ is used to treat metastatic renal cell carcinoma and melanoma.

5. _____ helps prevent infection by decreasing the incidence, severity, and duration of neutropenia associated with chemotherapy.

6. _____ _____ _____ is used to treat adults with genital warts.

7. _____ is an interferon beta-1a used to treat multiple sclerosis.

8. _____ agents increase the effects of interferons.

9. _____ decrease the effects of aldesleukin.

10. Acute, flu-like symptoms are more likely to occur with _____.

■ Clinical Challenge

A client is taking interferon alfa-2a for hairy cell leukemia. He has been discharged from the hospital. A caregiver will administer the injections. Why is it important that the medication be administered as prescribed? What would the nurse stress to the caregiver concerning this medication?

■ Review Questions

1. The nurse should be aware that immunostimulant therapy:
   a. should be administered by mouth
   b. involves shaking the medication vigorously before preparing the administration
   c. has very few minor adverse effects
   d. may lead to noncompliance in clients

2. Your client is receiving darbepoetin alfa (Aranesp) for anemia associated with chronic renal failure. You will omit a dose if the hemoglobin level is:
   a. >2 g/dL
   b. >5 g/dL
   c. >8 g/dL
   d. >12 g/dL

3. A client is being treated with aldesleukin (Proleukin) for metastatic renal cell carcinoma. He has just experienced a severe reaction from the medication. You suspect that his physician will:
   a. decrease the dosage of the drug
   b. withhold one or more doses
   c. add a second drug to decrease adverse effect
   d. continue with prescribed dosage and see whether reaction occurs again

4. Interferons should be taken:
   a. in the morning
   b. at 12 noon
   c. with the evening meal
   d. at bedtime

5. Your client has neutropenia as a result of chemotherapy. In order to prevent infection, pegfilgrastim (Neulasta) will be started:
   a. immediately after the last dose of chemotherapy
   b. 24 hours after the last dose of chemotherapy
   c. in between chemotherapy doses
   d. 2 weeks after chemotherapy has ended

6. Aldesleukin is contraindicated in clients with preexisting:
   a. diabetes mellitus
   b. Parkinson's disease
   c. spastic colon or diverticulitis
   d. cardiovascular or pulmonary disease

7. Oprelvekin (Neumega) is being given to your 7-year-old client who has thrombocytopenia. You will observe for which of the following adverse effects?
   a. hypertension
   b. bradycardia
   c. tachycardia
   d. hypotension

8. You are aware that your client had a preexisting renal impairment before she started sargramostim therapy. You will monitor which of the following?
   a. serum creatinine levels
   b. electrolyte levels
   c. blood glucose levels
   d. aspartate transaminase levels

9. Your 78-year-old client is taking oprelvekin (Neumega). Which of the following adverse effects is most likely to occur in your client?

   a. bone pain

   b. atrial dysrhythmias

   c. increased uric acid

   d. arthralgias levels

10. A favorable outcome for a client who is on epoetin alfa therapy would be:

    a. increase in hematocrit

    b. decrease in hemoglobin

    c. increase in white blood cells

    d. decrease in red blood cells

CHAPTER 36

Corticosteroids and Immunosuppressants

■ Exercises

Match the following.

1. ____ mycophenolate

2. ____ cyclosporine (Sandimmune)

3. ____ lymphocyte immune globulin (Atgam)

4. ____ etanercept (Enbrel)

5. ____ azathioprine (Imuran)

6. ____ tacrolimus (Prograf)

7. ____ basiliximab (Simulect)

8. ____ methotrexate (Rheumatrex)

9. ____ infliximab (Remicade)

10. ____ sirolimus

a. Insoluble in water, formulated in alcohol, olive oil, and castor oil

b. Used to prevent renal transplant rejection

c. A folate antagonist used in the treatment of cancer and severe arthritis

d. Obtained from the serum of horses immunized with human thymus tissue or lymphocytes

e. A monoclonal antibody used to treat rheumatoid arthritis and Crohn's disease

f. Used for prevention and treatment of rejection reactions with kidney, heart, and liver transplantations

g. Children require higher doses to maintain plasma drug levels

h. A tumor necrosis factor receptor used to treat rheumatoid arthritis when other treatments have failed

i. Given in combination with cyclosporine or corticosteroid to people receiving renal transplant

j. Antimetabolite that interferes with production of RNA and DNA

Place a T (true) or F (false) in each blank.

1. ____ The immune response is normally a protective mechanism that helps the body defend itself.

2. ____ The largest amount of glucocorticoids are produced during the evening hours.

3. ____ The most expected adverse effect of corticosteroids is increased risk of infection.

4. ____ Corticosteroids increase the formation and function of antibodies.

5. ____ Patients on long-term immunosuppressant drug therapy are at increased risk of cancer.

6. ____ Adrenal insufficiency is an indication for corticosteroid use.

7. ____ Corticosteroids decrease the effects of adrenergic bronchodilators.

8. ____ Corticosteroids have anticancer effects in hematologic malignancies.

9. ____ Oral contraceptives may decrease the effect of prednisolone.

10. ____ During periods of stress, corticosteroid therapy must be increased.

▪Clinical Challenge

Your client has been diagnosed with primary adrenocortical insufficiency (Addison's disease) due to cancer. Outline your teaching plan related to replacement therapy. How will the diagnosis of cancer affect your plan?

An 81-year-old male has a diagnosis of severe rheumatoid arthritis and has had a progressive treatment regimen of prednisone, methotrexate, infliximab (Remicade), and leflunomide (Arava). During a clinical treatment of Remicade, he and his wife voice concern about adverse effects of all the medication he is taking. How should the nurse respond?

▪Review Questions

1. Which of the following would be the most appropriate nursing diagnosis for a client taking steroids?
   a. imbalanced nutrition: less than body requirements
   b. deficient fluid volume
   c. risk for infection
   d. ineffective breathing pattern

2. Your client has been on an oral corticosteroid for 3 weeks. He tells you that he has missed several doses. An appropriate response to him would be:
   a. "Don't worry about it. It will not affect the intended outcome."
   b. "Alteration in administration of the drug can cause complications."
   c. "Next time you miss a dose, take an extra tablet with the next dose."
   d. "You really should be more careful in taking your medication."

3. Your client has a diagnosis of adrenocortical insufficiency and is steroid dependent. She has just lost her husband in a motor vehicle accident. During this time of stress, her medication will be:
   a. the same
   b. decreased
   c. increased
   d. discontinued

4. Clients on long-term immunosuppressant drug therapy with autoimmune disorders and organ transplantation are at increased risk for:
   a. hypotension
   b. osteoporosis
   c. cancer
   d. chronic urinary tract infections

5. Before a client is put on cyclosporine (Sandimmune) to help prevent a rejection reaction from a liver transplant, the nurse should assess for which of the following?
   a. use of alcohol
   b. weight loss
   c. blood glucose level
   d. activity level

6. Sirolimus (Rapamune) is given in combination with cyclosporine (Sandimmune) to prevent renal transplant rejection. The two drugs given 4 hours apart have a greater total effect than the sum of their individual effects. This drug action is:
   a. synergism
   b. simple summation
   c. potentiation
   d. antagonism

7. Which of the following elevated lab results could indicate hepatotoxicity from the use of cyclosporine (Sandimmune)?

   a. serum aminotransferases and bilirubin

   b. blood glucose level and ketone count

   c. urine specify gravity and urine pH

   d. arterial blood gases and O_2 saturation

8. The nurse will encourage the client to take which of the following medications at a different time rather than with the prescribed corticosteroid?

   a. Ampicillin

   b. Mylanta

   c. Advil

   d. Dramamine

9. You are preparing an oral dose of cyclosporine (Sandimmune) for your client. You will mix the medication with:

   a. room-temperature apple juice

   b. cold orange juice

   c. lukewarm grapefruit juice

   d. cold milk

10. Your client, age 53, has severe asthma. She has taken prednisone (Deltasone) for years. Recently, her physician has started her on alternate-day therapy. She tells you she would rather take her medication every day. Which of the following would be your best response?

   a. "This schedule will be more convenient for you."

   b. "This schedule will enable you to lose weight."

   c. "This schedule will decrease the cost of your medication."

   d. "This schedule allows rest periods so that adverse effects are decreased but the anti-inflammatory effects continue."

CHAPTER 37

Bronchodilating and Other Antiasthmatic Drugs

■ Exercises

Place a T (true) or F (false) in each blank.

1. ____ Hispanics have a higher death rate from asthma than do other ethnic groups.

2. ____ Children who are exposed to tobacco smoke are at risk for the development of asthma.

3. ____ A chronic cough can be the only symptom of asthma.

4. ____ Asthma is a respiratory disorder characterized by bronchodilation.

5. ____ Anti-asthmatic medications can increase acid reflux.

6. ____ Anti-inflammatory drugs reduce inflammation by increasing bronchoconstriction.

7. ____ Adrenergic bronchodilators are contraindicated in clients with severe cardiac disease.

8. ____ Epinephrine is the treatment of choice to relieve acute asthma.

9. ____ IV administration of a corticosteroid in acute severe asthma has a therapeutic advantage over oral administration.

10. ____ Leukotriene modifiers are effective in relieving acute attacks of asthma.

Fill in the blank.

1. _____ and _____ are used only for prophylaxis of acute bronchoconstriction.

2. _____ is used to prevent exercise-induced asthma.

3. Muscle tremor is the most frequent adverse effect of _____.

4. _____, an anticholinergic agent, is available in a nasal spray to treat rhinorrhea associated with allergic rhinitis and the common cold.

5. _____ therapy is contraindicated in clients with acute gastritis and peptic ulcer disease.

6. _____ are chemical mediators of bronchoconstriction and inflammation.

7. _____ is contraindicated in clients with liver disease.

8. _____ and _____ prevent the release of bronchoconstrictive and inflammatory substances when mast cells are confronted with allergens.

9. _____ is a selective beta-2 adrenergic agonist that is a long-acting bronchodilator.

10. With chronic asthma, a _____ is usually taken by inhalation on a daily basis.

▪ Clinical Challenge

Your client is a 15-year-old girl who has asthma. She has a short-acting bronchodilator inhaler albuterol (Proventil); however, she states that it "doesn't seem to help." How do you respond?

You determine she is not using the inhaler correctly. What do you do?

You notice that she has difficulty in manually holding and operating the inhaler. What do you recommend?

▪ Review Questions

1. A 16-year-old enters the hospital emergency room with a severe asthma attack. Which of the following drugs will most likely be used?

   a. salmeterol

   b. epinephrine

   c. albuterol

   d. formoterol

2. Your asthmatic client's medication has been changed to theophylline (Theo-Dur). Which of the following is most important to include in his client teaching?

   a. Take only on an empty stomach.

   b. Increase intake of fatty foods.

   c. Decrease intake of fluids.

   d. Limit intake of caffeine.

3. When teaching an asthma client the proper technique for administering a metered-dose inhaler, the nurse will emphasize:

   a. not to eat or drink prior to or after administration

   b. to lie in semi-Fowler's position while administering the inhaler

   c. to hold his breath for 10 seconds after inhaling the medication before exhaling

   d. to place his lips firmly around the inhaler's mouthpiece

4. Your client has been diagnosed with asthma. You have just finished explaining the use of a metered-dose inhaler. Which of the following responses indicates the need for further instruction?

   a. "I should inhale deeply before depressing the inhaler."

   b. "I will shake the inhaler well before each use."

   c. "I will wait about 5 minutes before I inhale for the second time."

   d. "I will not use more than one or two puffs per treatment."

5. Your client has been using a beclomethasone (Beclovent) inhaler for several months. She is in the clinic complaining of a rash in her mouth. She is upset and states she knows it is from the inhaler she is using. Which of the following should you do?

   a. Recommend that she stop using the Beclovent inhaler immediately.

   b. Instruct your client to decrease the dosage of Beclovent.

   c. Inform her that she is having an allergic reaction to something she has eaten.

   d. Remind her that she must rinse her mouth after each treatment.

6. Your client has been taking zafirlukast (Accolate) for asthma for 3 weeks. She is in the clinic for a follow-up visit. Which of the following findings would cause you alarm?

   a. pulse rate of 84

   b. absence of wheezing

   c. pink nail beds

   d. whites of eyes are yellow in color

7. A client who is on theophylline (Theo-Dur) is in the clinic for a theophylline level. You know that the optimal therapeutic range for this drug is:

   a. 0.5 to 5 mcg/mL

   b. 10 to 20 mcg/mL

   c. 20 to 30 mcg/mL

   d. 50 to 65 mcg/mL

8. Which of the following drugs is used only for prophylaxis of bronchoconstriction?

    a. epinephrine

    b. salmeterol

    c. isoproterenol

    d. albuterol

9. Your client is taking a combination of ipratropium and albuterol (Combivent). Which of the following will you stress as a common adverse effect?

    a. increased pulse rate

    b. rhinorrhea

    c. weight gain

    d. cough

10. You are instructing your client on the administration of zafirlukast (Accolate). Which of the following should you include in your instructions?

    a. Take 1 hour before or 2 hours after a meal.

    b. Take with fatty foods.

    c. Take medication once daily.

    d. May be taken with or without food.

CHAPTER 38

Antihistamines

■ Exercises

Answer the following.

1. Where is histamine mainly located in the body?

2. What causes histamine to be discharged from mast cells and basophils?

3. Where are H_1 receptors located?

4. List six responses that may occur when histamine binds with H_1 receptors.

5. List three responses that occur when H_2 receptors are stimulated.

Match the following.

1. _____ type I allergic reaction

2. _____ urticaria

3. _____ epinephrine

4. _____ anaphylaxis

5. _____ hydroxyzine (Atarax)

6. _____ serum sickness

7. _____ allergic rhinitis

8. _____ antigens

9. _____ anaphylactoid reactions

10. _____ type II allergic reaction

a. Mediated by IgG and IgM

b. Drug of choice for treating severe anaphylaxis

c. A vascular reaction of the skin characterized by papules or wheals and severe itching

d. Example of type I allergic reaction

e. Foreign materials (environmental or ingested substances)

f. Prescribed for pruritus

g. A delayed hypersensitivity reaction most often caused by drugs

h. Inflammation of nasal mucosa

i. May occur on first exposure to a foreign substance

j. Mediated by IgE

■ Clinical Challenge

Your client, a 65-year-old female, has been prescribed cetirizine (Zyrtec) to treat her seasonal allergies. What assessment data do you need in order to provide client education concerning use of an antihistamine?

■ Review Questions

1. A 25-year-old female calls the clinic at 3:00 PM and tells you she forgot to take her morning dose of fexofenadine (Allegra). She wants to know what she should do. You tell her to:

   a. double her evening dose

   b. skip the evening dose and start back in the morning

   c. forget about the morning dose and take the evening dose early

   d. take the morning dose now and the evening dose at the scheduled time

2. Your client has just been placed on an antihistamine for allergic rhinitis. Which of the following will you be sure to include in your teaching plan regarding antihistamines?

   a. Use sunscreen outdoors.

   b. Weigh daily and note any change in weight.

   c. Reduce fat intake in diet.

   d. Reduce intake of citrus juices.

3. A 32-year-old businessman is in the clinic for allergies. He has to make a major presentation in 3 days, and his allergies are worse. He asks whether the doctor can prescribe another antihistamine for him to use with the loratadine (Claritin) he is already taking. Your best response to him would be:

   a. "Sure, I'll ask right now."

   b. "If you take another antihistamine, you will have to decrease the Claritin dosage."

   c. "You should not take two antihistamines at the same time because of possible severe adverse effects."

   d. "Why do you think you need more medication?"

4. A 22-year-old male is in the clinic for seasonal allergies. He states that he works in construction and operates heavy equipment. Which of the following drugs will be prescribed for him?

   a. desloratadine (Clarinex)

   b. hydroxyzine (Vistaril)

   c. promethazine (Phenergan)

   d. chlorpheniramine (Chlor-Trimeton)

5. Antihistamines may be contraindicated for people with:

   a. diabetes mellitus

   b. urinary retention

   c. Alzheimer's disease

   d. multiple sclerosis

6. Your client is taking diphenhydramine (Benadryl) for allergic rhinitis. Which of the following nursing diagnoses would be appropriate, especially during the first few days of therapy?

   a. deficient knowledge: safe and accurate drug use

   b. risk for injury related to drowsiness

   c. deficient knowledge: strategies for minimizing exposure to allergens

   d. risk for activity intolerance related to antihistamine

7. On a return visit to the clinic, your client, a 69-year-old male, complains of difficulty voiding. He was seen 1 week ago for pruritus. You suspect he may have:

   a. prostatic hypertrophy

   b. renal failure

   c. diabetes mellitus

   d. cardiac dysrhythmias

8. Which of the following antihistamines is not recommended for children with chickenpox or flu-like infections?

   a. hydroxyzine (Atarax)

   b. clemastine (Tavist)

   c. chlorpheniramine (Chlor-Trimeton)

   d. diphenhydramine (Benadryl)

9. Your client is to begin taking loratadine (Claritin). She asks you how long will it take to help her allergies. Your response should be:

a. "You should feel better immediately."

b. "You should see some effects within 1 to 3 hours of your first dose."

c. "It will take about 3 weeks before you will see any effects."

d. "In about 2 days, you should feel better."

10. When instructing your client in taking loratadine (Claritin), you should include which of the following?

a. Take on an empty stomach.

b. Chew the tablet and follow with a glass of water.

c. Take with meals.

d. Take three times a day.

Drug Therapy of Heart Failure

■ Exercises

Define the following.

1. Heart failure

2. Endothelin

3. Digitalization

Place T (true) or F (false) in each blank.

1. ____ Clients with atrial fibrillation exhibit dyspnea and fatigue at rest.

2. ____ Digoxin toxicity may occur at any serum level.

3. ____ Digoxin is the drug of choice for clients with acute myocardial infarction.

4. ____ The onset of action for oral digoxin is 30 minutes to 2 hours.

5. ____ Yellow-green vision is an adverse effect of digoxin.

6. ____ The drug of choice for acute heart failure is an angiotensin-converting enzyme (ACE) inhibitor.

7. ____ In chronic heart failure, there is a high risk for hypokalemia.

8. ____ Digoxin dosage must be reduced by approximately half in clients with renal failure.

9. ____ In the management of digoxin toxicity, potassium chloride may be given if the serum potassium level is low.

10 ____ In children, there is a significant difference between a therapeutic dose and a toxic dose.

11. ____ Digoxin toxicity develops more often and lasts longer in renal impairment.

12. ____ Hepatic impairment has a tremendous effect on digoxin clearance, and dosage adjustments must be made.

13. ____ Ephedra may be used by clients with heart failure.

14. ____ A client may substitute the brand and type of digoxin.

15. ____ In atrial fibrillation, digoxin slows the heart beat.

Match the following.

1. ____ thrombocytopenia

2. ____ lidocaine

3. ____ bosentan (Tracleer)

4. ____ nesiritide

5. ____ digoxin

6. ____ atropine

7. ____ photophobia

8. ____ furosemide

9. ____ pulmonary edema

10. ____ cough

a. A loop diuretic used in clients with heart failure who have impaired renal function

b. Occurs when left ventricular failure causes blood to accumulate in pulmonary veins and tissues

c. An endothelin receptor antagonist used to treat pulmonary hypertension

d. The only commonly used digitalis glycoside

e. An adverse effect of prolonged use of inamrinone

f. A characteristic of moderate or severe heart failure

g. An antiarrhythmic local anesthetic agent used to decrease myocardial irritability

h. Used in the management of acute heart failure to increase diuresis and secretion of sodium and decrease the secretion of neurohormones

i. Used in the management of bradycardia

j. An adverse effect of digoxin

■ Clinical Challenge

A client, a 70-year-old female, is admitted to the coronary care unit complaining of nausea and vomiting. She has a heart rate of 46 beats per minute. Initial assessment reveals that she is currently taking digoxin, furosemide, and a potassium supplement. A diagnosis of digoxin toxicity is made according to serum digoxin concentrations. With this diagnosis, what will the nurse monitor throughout the client's stay in the unit? What is the therapeutic range of digoxin the nurse will be looking for?

After several days in the unit, the client's serum digoxin is within the therapeutic range. She is to be discharged on Lanoxin 0.125 mg PO daily. What will the nurse include in client instruction regarding the medication?

The client asks the nurse why her heart rate was so slow. How should the nurse respond?

■ Review Questions

1. Your client has been successfully digitalized. Serum levels of digoxin are within therapeutic range. The nurse will monitor which of the following to determine the maintenance dose of digoxin?

   a. hepatic function

   b. creatinine clearance

   c. potassium levels

   d. magnesium levels

2. A 72-year-old male is admitted to the cardiac care unit with severe heart failure. He is to receive a bolus dose of inamirone (Inacor). The nurse will observe for which of the following adverse effects?

   a. dysrhythmias

   b. headache

   c. disorientation

   d. seizures

3. A client is to be discharged on Lanoxin 0.125 mg daily. Which of the following statements by the client indicates successful client teaching by the nurse?

   a. "If I miss a dose, I should not take 2 tablets in 1 day."

   b. "I will have to take this drug 2 or 3 months."

   c. "This drug can cause a bitter taste in my mouth."

   d. "This drug may cause me to retain fluid."

4. The nurse is monitoring a client's serum digoxin levels and is aware that the therapeutic range is:

   a. 0.125 to 0.5 ng/mL

   b. 0.2 to 1.0 ng/mL

   c. 0.5 to 2.0 ng/mL

   d. 3.5 to 5.0 ng/mL

5. A nursing action related to the care of a client who is receiving digoxin includes:

   a. administering the drug subcutaneously

   b. relying on client blood pressure readings for dosage

   c. reporting an apical heart rate below 60 to the client's physician

   d. discontinuing the medication if the serum digoxin level is within therapeutic range

6. A 58-year-old male is admitted to the emergency room. A diagnosis of severe digoxin toxicity is made. Which of the following drugs may be given immediately?

   a. digoxin immune fab

   b. furosemide

   c. captopril

   d. dopamine

7. Your client is taking digoxin (Lanoxin) 0.125 mg daily for heart failure. She reports to you that since she has been on the drug, she can breathe better and her heart rate has been around 74 beats per minute. You also notice that, according to the scales, she has lost 3 pounds since her last visit. You suspect that:

   a. the drug dosage will be increased

   b. the drug dosage will stay the same

   c. the drug dosage will be decreased

   d. the drug will be discontinued

8. Which of the following should be emphasized when instructing a client who is to begin taking digoxin (Lanoxin)?

   a. Digoxin tablets may be crushed and taken with food.

   b. Digoxin should not be taken with an antacid.

   c. It doesn't matter what time of day digoxin is taken.

   d. If a daily dose is missed, it may be taken with the next dose.

9. Which of the following indicates a therapeutic effect of digoxin (Lanoxin) when given for an atrial dsyrhythmia?

   a. increase in weight

   b. elimination of pulse deficit

   c. gradual increase in heart rate

   d. decrease in edema

10. Your client is to receive nesiritide (Natrecor) for acute heart failure. It is important for the nurse to remember that:

    a. the drug must be administered through a separate IV line

    b. a bolus injection of Natrecor must be given over a 10-minute period

    c. the drug cannot be diluted with sodium chloride

    d. it is not necessary to prime the infusion tubing prior to administration

CHAPTER 40

Antidysrhythmic Drugs

■ Exercises

Fill in the blank.

1. Electrical impulses in the heart depend on the movement of _____ and _____ ions into a myocardial cell and movement of _____ ions out of the cell.

2. The ability of a cardiac muscle cell to respond to an electrical stimulus is called _____.

3. The period following contraction when the cell cannot respond to a new stimulus is called the _____ _____ period.

4. The period before the resting membrane potential is reached and a stimulus greater than normal is needed to produce a response is called _____ _____ period.

5. _____ is the ability of cardiac tissue to transmit electrical impulses.

6. Cardiac dysrhythmias result from _____ in electrical impulses.

7. _____ increases myocardial irritability and is considered a risk factor for atrial and ventricular dysrhythmias.

8. _____ _____ is the most common dysrhythmia.

9. _____ is the only FDA-approved antidysrhythmic drug for children.

10. _____ _____ are the most common sustained dysrhythmias in children.

Match the following.

1. ____ tocainide (Tonocard)

2. ____ flecainide (Tambocor)

3. ____ lidocaine (Xylocaine)

4. ____ sotalol (Betapace)

5. ____ ibutilide (Corvert)

6. ____ phenytoin (Dilantin)

7. ____ quinidine (Quinaglute)

8. ____ amiodarone (Cordarone)

9. ____ procainamide (Pronestyl)

10 ____ acebutolol (Sectral)

a. When used long term, may increase the effects of anticoagulants

b. Prototype of class IB antidysrhythmias; must be given by injection

c. Contraindicated in clients with asthma

d. Anticonvulsant used to treat dysrhythmias

e. Indicated for recent onset of atrial fibrillation or atrial flutter

f. Can be used to terminate supraventricular tachy-dysrhythmias

g. Prototype for class IA antidysrhythmias; use is declining

h. Used for chronic therapy to prevent ventricular dysrhythmias precipitated by exercise

i. Recommended for use only in life-threatening ventricular dysrhythmias

j. Oral analog of lidocaine

■ Clinical Challenge

A 79-year-old client is admitted to the emergency room with severe chest pain. He is diaphoretic and complaining of shortness of breath and nausea. The cardiac monitor reveals sinus tachycardia and frequent premature ventricular complexes. He is to receive an IV lidocaine bolus. How much lidocaine will the nurse prepare? How will the medication be administered? After the bolus dose, the nurse will maintain a continuous infusion of lidocaine at what rate? How will the nurse monitor the lidocaine levels?

What does the nurse need to know about mixing other drugs with lidocaine? What side effects will the nurse observe for?

■ Review Questions

1. A client has been diagnosed with ventricular tachycardia. He is started on tocainide (Tono-card). The nurse will assess for which of the following?
   a. headache
   b. diarrhea
   c. nausea
   d. muscle and joint pain

2. Your client is to receive disopyramide (Nor-pace). The nurse should assess for which of the following conditions?
   a. hepatic disease
   b. peptic ulcer disease
   c. seizure disorder
   d. renal insufficiency

3. The expected outcome for a client who is taking an antidysrhythmic drug would be:
   a. increased cardiac output
   b. decreased cardiac output
   c. increased renal insufficiency
   d. decreased respiratory distress

4. Your client is being discharged from the hospital on an antidysrhythmic drug. It is important that the client/caregiver report which of the following?
   a. dizziness
   b. constipation
   c. increased appetite
   d. stiffness in joints

5. Before administering an antidysrhythmic drug, the nurse should:
   a. take the client's temperature
   b. assess the client's mental status
   c. check the apical and radial pulses
   d. place the client in semi-Fowler's position

6. Your client has been on disopyramide (Norpace) for 3 days. You will assess for which of the following adverse effects?
   a. increased blood pressure
   b. dry mouth
   c. edema
   d. severe diarrhea

7. The heart monitor indicates that your client is experiencing supraventricular tachycardia. You are to administer diltiazem (Cardizem) 20 mg IV push. During the administration of this drug you will observe for:
   a. decreased heart rate
   b. increased heart rate
   c. increased blood pressure
   d. increased body temperature

8. Verapamil (Calan) is contraindicated in a client who has:
   a. diabetes mellitus
   b. respiratory impairment
   c. digoxin toxicity
   d. edema

9. Which of the following instructions should be given to a client who is taking quinidine (Quinaglute)?

    a. Decrease salt intake.

    b. Take the medication with orange juice.

    c. Decrease the fiber in diet.

    d. Take the medication with meals.

10. Which of the following is the most commonly used antidysrhythmic drug used in children?

    a. propranolol (Inderal)

    b. ibutilide (Corvet)

    c. dofetilide (Tikosyn)

    d. esmolol (Brevibloc)

■Cardiac Electrophysiology Diagram

Fill in the blanks in Figure 40-1 with the terms below to identify the components of the heart's conduction system.

AV junction
Purkinje fibers
Inferior branch of left
  bundle branch
SA node

Anterior branch of left
  bundle branch
Bundle of His
AV node

Main stem of left
  bundle branch
Internodal tracts
Right bundle branch
Intra-atrial tract

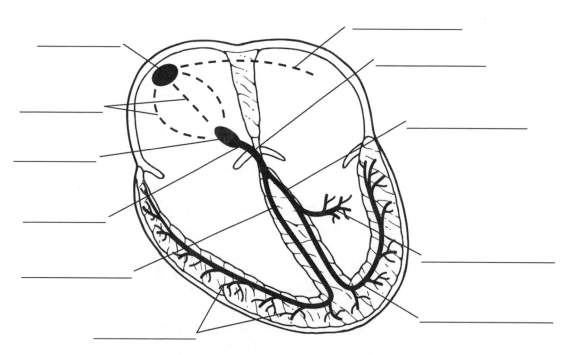

FIGURE 40.1

■Dysrhythmia Analysis

Select the appropriate term from the list below to pair each of the dysrhythmias with a drug that might be ordered for its treatment.

Digoxin (Lanoxin)   Atrial fibrillation
Lidocaine (Xylocaine)   Sinus bradycardia
Supraventricular tachycardia   Atropine
Adenosine (Adenocard)   Premature ventricular contractions

1. Dysrhythmia _____ Treatment _____

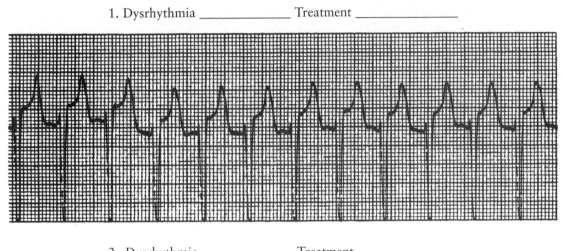

2. Dysrhythmia _____ Treatment _____

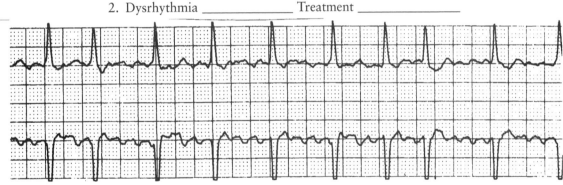

3. Dysrhythmia _____ Treatment _____

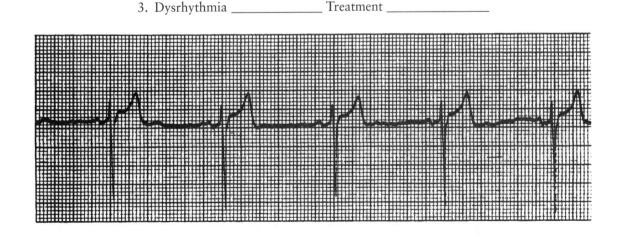

4. Dysrhythmia _____ Treatment _____

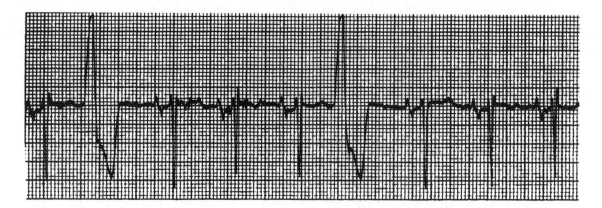

CHAPTER 41

Antianginal Drugs

■ Exercises

Answer the following.

1. What causes angina pectoris to develop?

2. Describe the development of coronary artery disease.

3. List the three main types of angina.

4. Describe anginal pain.

5. List the drugs used for myocardial ischemia.

Match the following.

1. ____ Beta-adrenergic blocking agents

2. ____ nifedipine (Procardia)

3. ____ nadolol (Corgard)

4. ____ aspirin

5. ____ nitroglycerin

6. ____ cimetidine

7. ____ isosorbide mononitrate (Ismo)

8. ____ carbamazepine (Tegretol)

9. ____ propranolol (Inderal)

10. ____ isosorbide dinitrate (Isordil)

a. The prototype beta blocker

b. Organic nitrate prototype

c. Used in long-term management of angina to decrease frequency and severity of attacks

d. Has become part of the standard of care in coronary heart disease

e. Beta-adrenergic blocker that can be given once daily

f. Used only for prophylaxis of angina

g. Acts mainly on vascular smooth muscle to produce vasodilation

h. Decreases effects of calcium channel blockers

i. Effective oral dose obtained by increasing the dose until headache occurs

j. Increases beta-blocking effect of propranolol

Place a T (true) or F (false) in each blank.

1. ____ The most common causes of angina are low blood pressure and an increased amount of blood and oxygen to the heart.

2. ____ Long-acting medications for angina are not effective in relieving sudden anginal pain.

3. ____ Clients may increase or decrease dosages of medication for angina according to frequency and severity of attacks.

4. ____ Nitroglycerin tablets should be replaced every 6 months.

5. ____ Hypertension is an adverse effect of antianginal drugs.

6. ____ Nitroglycerin patches should be applied at the same time each day.

7. ____ Nitroglycerin patches may be applied anywhere on the body.

8. ____ It takes between 3 and 5 hours for transmucosal tablets to dissolve.

9. ____ Bradycardia is an adverse effect of nitrates.

10. ____ Nifedipine (Procardia) may cause hypotension.

■ Clinical Challenge

The client is a 43-year-old male who is admitted to the hospital with increasing episodes of angina with minimal exertion. He is to begin isosorbide dinitrate sustained-release 40-mg tablets. What would be the nurse's instructions regarding administration of this drug?

The client shows no improvement in 12 hours. The physician orders nifedipine (Procardia) 10 mg PO every 6 hours. Why will the nurse monitor the client for hypotension?

The client begins to show improvement and is ready for discharge. What instructions will the nurse give to the client?

■ Review Questions

1. Your client is admitted to the hospital with a diagnosis of chest pain. He has an order for nitroglycerin 0.3 mg SL PRN for chest pain. Which of the following actions should you do when he complains of chest pain?

   a. Call the physician.

   b. Place 3 nitroglycerin tablets under his tongue.

   c. Have the client swallow a tablet every 5 minutes for 20 minutes.

   d. Administer a tablet under his tongue; may need to repeat in 5 minutes and again in 5 more minutes.

2. Which of the following would indicate a contraindication for the use of nitroglycerin?

   a. a client with hypertension

   b. a client with severe anemia

   c. a client with thyroid disease

   d. a client with diabetes mellitus

3. An expected outcome for a client who has just taken nitroglycerin should be:

   a. increased pulse

   b. decreased pulse

   c. increased blood pressure

   d. decreased blood pressure

4. Which of the following drugs is used for prophylaxis of angina?

   a. nitroglycerin

   b. isosorbide mononitrate

   c. propranolol

   d. nifedipine

5. The most common adverse effect of nitroglycerin is:
   a. diuresis
   b. pounding headache
   c. irritability
   d. dry mouth

6. Which of the following conditions would a
   nurse assess for before starting nifedipine (Procardia) therapy?
   a. severe hepatic disease
   b. Raynaud's syndrome
   c. diabetes mellitus
   d. myasthenia gravis

7. Your client complains of headaches and dizziness with nitrate therapy. Which of the following would be the most appropriate response to
   her?
   a. "Avoid strenuous activity and stand up
      slowly."
   b. "These effects are temporary and should
      subside with continuous use."
   c. "You will have these adverse effects as long
      as you use nitroglycerin."
   d. "You may reduce your dosage to help relieve
      the adverse effects."

8. Your client is taking a calcium channel blocker.
   He should avoid over-the-counter medications
   containing:
   a. ephedrine
   b. acetaminophen
   c. calcium
   d. iron

9. In regard to the administration of oral nitrates,
   the nurse will instruct the client to:
   a. take on any empty stomach
   b. take with food
   c. place the tablet between the cheek and gum
   d. place the tablet under the tongue

10. You are applying a topical preparation of nitro-
    glycerin. Your *initial* action will be to:
    a. place the ointment on a nonhairy part of the
       body
    b. wipe off the previous dose
    c. cover the area with a plastic wrap or tape
    d. put on a pair of gloves

CHAPTER 42

Drugs Used in Hypotension and Shock

■ Exercises

Match the following.

1. ____ septic shock

2. ____ hypovolemic shock

3. ____ anaphylactic shock

4. ____ neurogenic shock

5. ____ distributive shock

6. ____ cardiogenic shock

a. Can result from any organisms that enter the bloodstream

b. Results from hypersensitivity

c. Characterized by severe vasodilation, which results in severe hypotension and impairment of blood flow

d. Results from inadequate sympathetic nervous system stimulation

e. Involves a loss of intravascular fluid volume

f. Occurs when the myocardium has lost its ability to contract efficiently and maintain adequate cardiac output

Fill in the blank.

1. Drugs used in the management of shock are primarily _____ drugs.

2. _____ is a naturally occurring catecholamine that is useful in hypovolemic and cardiogenic shock.

3. _____ is the drug of choice for management of anaphylactic shock.

4. _____ is used only in shock associated with decreased heart rates and myocardial depression.

5. _____ is used mainly in hypotension occurring from spinal anesthesia.

6. _____ is used mainly in clients who do not respond to dopamine or dobutamine.

7. _____ and _____ are most often the cardiotonic drugs used in critically ill clients.

8. _____ is the drug of first choice in distributive shock.

9. _____ is less likely to cause tachycardia and dysrhythmias than are dopamine and isoproterenol.

10. _____ decreases the effectiveness of dopamine.

■ Clinical Challenge

Your client is in the cardiac care unit with a diagnosis of cardiogenic shock. He is getting dopamine (Intropin) intravenously. What will dopamine do for this client? Why is adequate fluid therapy necessary for this client?

■ Review Questions

1. You are starting an IV on a client who is to receive IV dopamine (Intropin). To decrease the risk of extravasation, you will:

   a. administer a concentrated solution of dopamine

   b. dilute the dopamine in 50 mL of IV fluids

   c. use a large vein for the venipuncture site

   d. mix the dopamine with other drugs to be administered

2. You have started an IV dopamine (Intropin) drip. The flow rate will be titrated according to:

   a. the client's response to the drug

   b. the manufacturer's directions

   c. the weight of the client

   d. the type of shock the client is experiencing

3. Your client has been receiving dopamine (Intropin) for the management of hypovolemia. The physician has discontinued the drug. You will stop the drug gradually in order to prevent:

   a. hypertension

   b. hypotension

   c. dysrhythmia

   d. tachycardia

4. An expected client outcome of drug therapy for hypotension associated with shock is:

   a. systolic blood pressure of 180 and heart rate of 40

   b. systolic blood pressure of 80 and heart rate of 120

   c. systolic blood pressure of 98 and heart rate of 70

   d. systolic blood pressure of 130 and heart rate of 50

5. Extravasation of metaraminol (Aramine) has occurred with your client. Which of the following drugs will you administer?

   a. diltiazem (Cardizem)

   b. phentolamine (Regitine)

   c. cinoxacin (Cinobac)

   d. betamethasone (Celestone)

6. Which of the following is the most important nursing measure when caring for a client who is being managed for shock?

   a. Monitor blood pressure frequently.

   b. Take apical pulse prior to medication administration.

   c. Weigh daily.

   d. Decrease fluid intake.

7. A client with anaphylactic shock presents to the Emergency Department. You administer epinephrine. Therapeutic effects should occur within:

   a. 1 to 3 minutes

   b. 5 to 10 minutes

   c. 10 to 15 minutes

   d. 20 to 30 minutes

8. Dopamine (Intropin) is being given to your client who is experiencing cardiogenic shock. Which of the following is necessary for a maximum therapeutic effect of the drug?

   a. administration of a cardiac glycoside

   b. a heart rate above 50

   c. an infusion rate of 100 µg/kg/min

   d. adequate fluid therapy

9. Which of the following decreases the effectiveness of vasopressor drugs?

   a. acidosis

   b. alkalosis

   c. benign prostatic hypertrophy

   d. hypokalemia

10. Your client is receiving isoproterenol (Isuprel) in the management of shock. You will be aware of the following adverse effect?

    a. bradycardia

    b. tachycardia

    c. hypotension

    d. acidosis

CHAPTER 43

Antihypertensive Drugs

■ Exercises

Place a T (true) or F (false) in each blank.

1. ____ Hypertension is defined as a systolic pressure above 160 mm Hg or a diastolic pressure above 100 mm Hg on more than one blood pressure measurement.

2. ____ It is best to lower blood pressure gradually.

3. ____ Captopril (Capoten) is recommended as a first-line agent for treating hypertension in diabetic clients.

4. ____ Angiotensin II receptor blockers are more likely to cause hyperkalemia than are angiotensin-converting enzyme (ACE) inhibitors.

5. ____ Vasodilator antihypertensive drugs directly relax smooth muscle in blood vessels to decrease peripheral vascular resistance.

6. ____ Increased blood pressure in children often leads to hypertension as young adults.

7. ____ Captopril (Capoten) is a first-line agent for children with hypertension.

8. ____ A diuretic is the drug of first choice in older adults and African Americans who are hypertensive.

9. ____ ACE inhibitors are used to help diabetic clients with renal impairment.

10. ____ Nonprescription medication may decrease the effectiveness of antihypertensive drugs.

Match the following

1. ____ captopril (Capoten)

2. ____ verapamil (Calan)

3. ____ nifedipine (Procardia)

4. ____ losartan (Cozaar)

5. ____ clonidine (Catapres)

6. ____ fenoldopam (Corlopam)

7. ____ hydrochlorothiazide

8. ____ prazosin (Minipress)

9. ____ sodium nitroprusside (Nipride)

10. ____ propranolol (Inderal)

a. Decreases renin release from the kidneys to decrease blood pressure

b. May cause orthostatic hypotension with palpitations

c. A short-acting calcium channel blocker used to treat hypertensive emergencies or urgencies

d. The first angiotensin II receptor blocker that may be used in combination with hydrochlorothiazide

e. A thiazide diuretic commonly used to treat hypertension

f. Serum thiocyanate levels should be monitored if drug is given longer than 72 hours

g. Initial dose may be taken at bedtime to prevent acute hypotension

h. A fast-acting drug indicated for short-term use in hypertensive emergencies

i. An alpha$_2$ receptor agonist that has delayed onset and is costly

j. A calcium channel blocker that dilates peripheral arteries and decreases peripheral vascular resistance by relaxing vascular smooth muscle to decrease blood pressure

■ Clinical Challenge

Your client, age 69, is admitted to the intensive care unit in hypertensive crisis. Her blood pressure at time of admission is 225/160 mm Hg. She is to receive nitroprusside (Nipride) IV. At what rate will you infuse the medication? What is the expected outcome of the Nipride therapy?

After a day of therapy, your client develops slurred speech and muscle twitching, and has a seizure. What should you do regarding Nipride therapy?

■ Review Questions

1. A client has been placed on captopril (Capoten) PO 25 mg BID. The nurse should instruct the client to:

   a. avoid citric juices with administration of the drug

   b. take the medication with a full glass of water

   c. take the medication on an empty stomach

   d. take the medication with food

2. Clonidine (Catapres) skin patches are applied to a hairless area on the upper arm or torso:

   a. every day

   b. every other day

   c. every 3 days

   d. every 7 days

3. The physician has prescribed prazosin (Minipress) 1 mg PO daily. When teaching the client about this drug, the nurse will stress:

   a. taking the first dose at bedtime to prevent dizziness

   b. limiting fluid intake to 1000 mL per day to decrease urinary output

   c. taking the drug early in the day to prevent sleepiness

   d. taking the drug on an empty stomach to promote absorption

4. The nurse is planning follow-up care for a client who has been taking hydrochlorothiazide (HydroDiuril) for hypertension. An additional antihypertensive agent has been added to her treatment regimen. The nurse is aware that:

   a. most clients on multidrug therapy follow the treatment plan

   b. most clients understand the importance of taking their medication as prescribed

   c. clients who are actively involved in their therapy are usually more compliant

   d. it is unusual for more than one medication to be prescribed for hypertension

5. In determining whether a client can be started on metoprolol (Lopressor), the nurse may question the client concerning:

   a. renal disease

   b. hepatic disease

   c. diabetes mellitus

   d. peptic ulcer disease

6. Your client has a prescription for benazepril (Lotensin). She asks you how long it will take to lower her blood pressure. The most appropriate response to her would be:

   a. "That's a question you should really ask your doctor."

   b. "It will probably take 3 to 4 weeks before you feel better."

   c. "This drug usually produces effects within 1 hour after you take the first dose."

   d. "It will take 6 months before you feel any effects of the drug."

7. Your client is diabetic and has been diagnosed with hypertension. An ACE inhibitor has been prescribed for her. Which of the following may develop as a result of the drug therapy?

   a. hypocalcemia

   b. hypercalcemia

   c. hypokalemia

   d. hyperkalemia

8. A 62-year-old female is taking losartan (Cozaar) for hypertension. It has been determined that the drug therapy is not controlling her blood pressure. Which of the following drugs may be added to her treatment plan?
   a. hydrochlorothiazide
   b. omeprazole
   c. fenoldopam
   d. nitroprusside

9. Chronic use of clonidine may result in:
   a. vertigo
   b. irritability
   c. nausea
   d. sodium and fluid retention

10. Your client is a 42-year-old African American male who has been diagnosed with hypertension. You suspect the doctor will initially prescribe:
    a. a calcium channel blocker
    b. a diuretic
    c. a beta blocker
    d. an ACE inhibitor

CHAPTER 44

Diuretics

■ Exercises

Fill in the blank.

1. The main function of the kidneys is to regulate the _____, _____, and _____ of body fluids.

2. The functional unit of the kidney is the _____.

3. Each nephron is composed of a _____ and a _____.

4. Most reabsorption occurs in the _____ _____.

5. _____ is the excessive accumulation of fluid in body tissues.

Match the following.

1. ____ spironolactone (Aldactone)

2. ____ hyperkalemia

3. ____ torsemide (Demadex)

4. ____ hydrochlorothiazide (HydroDIURIL)

5. ____ mannitol (Osmitrol)

6. ____ ototoxicity

7. ____ hypokalemia

8. ____ chlorothiazide (Diuril)

9. ____ pulmonary edema

10. ____ furosemide (Lasix)

a. An osmotic agent

b. Prototype for loop diuretics

c. May occur with potassium-losing diuretics

d. Adverse effect likely to occur with furosemide

e. Only thiazide diuretic that can be given IV

f. Adverse effect that occurs with osmotic diuretics

g. May be taken without regard to meals

h. Blocks the sodium-retaining effects of aldosterone

i. Major adverse effect of potassium-sparing diuretics

j. Most commonly used thiazide diuretic

Place a T (true) or F (false) in each blank.

1. ____ Diuretics decrease renal excretion of water, sodium, and other electrolytes.

2. ____ Each kidney contains approximately 100 nephrons.

3. ____ Sodium is reabsorbed in the ascending limb of Henle's loop.

4. ____ Edema interferes with blood flow to tissues.

5. ____ Initially, diuretics increase blood volume and cardiac output.

6. ____ Some diuretics may increase blood sugar levels.

7. ____ Dietary sodium is restricted in loop diuretic therapy.

8. ____ Loop diuretics are the drugs of choice when rapid diuresis is required.

9. ____ Furosemide (Lasix) is the loop diuretic most often used in children.

10. ____ There is an increased risk of hearing loss with the rapid administration of bumetanide (Bumex).

■ Clinical Challenge

Your client is admitted to the intensive care unit with symptoms of pulmonary edema and impaired renal function. IV furosemide (Lasix) is started. Because of the client's kidney disease, you will monitor which values? Which adverse effect will you also assess for?

Your client continues to improve and is discharged after several days. PO furosemide has been ordered. What will you include in your teaching plan when he is discharged?

■ Review Questions

1. A client is being treated for mild hypertension with chlorothiazide (Diuril) 500 mg PO daily. The nurse will teach her about which of the following adverse effects?

   a. muscle cramps

   b. drowsiness

   c. nausea and vomiting

   d. dry mouth

2. A 48-year-old female is diabetic and has been on oral hypoglycemics for several years. She has recently been diagnosed with hypertension and started on a thiazide diuretic. The nurse is aware that the diuretic may cause which of the following?

   a. hypoglycemia

   b. hyperglycemia

   c. hypokalemia

   d. hyperkalemia

3. The most appropriate nursing intervention for a client who is hospitalized and has just begun diuretic therapy would be to:

   a. record blood pressure readings two to four times daily

   b. weigh the client every other day

   c. record fluid intake and output every 36 hours

   d. enforce strict bedrest

4. To avoid increased risks of adverse effects, the nurse will administer an IV injection of furosemide over:

   a. 1 to 2 minutes

   b. 2 to 3 minutes

   c. 2 to 5 minutes

   d. 5 minutes

5. For clients at home, oral diuretics should be taken:

   a. early in the morning

   b. at noon

   c. during the afternoon hours

   d. at bedtime

6. Your client is taking an antihypertensive agent and a diuretic. You will teach him to:

   a. take both drugs on an empty stomach

   b. suck on hard candy

   c. change positions slowly

   d. increase daily exercise

7. A client is taking a potassium-sparing diuretic. Which of the following instructions should the nurse give to her?

   a. "Decrease salt in your diet."

   b. "Limit your intake of foods high in potassium."

   c. "Drink two glasses of orange juice and eat a banana every day."

   d. "Decrease fat in your diet."

8. A 16-year-old boy is admitted to the intensive care unit with increased intracranial pressure from a head injury. Which of the following diuretics will be administered to him?

   a. furosemide (Lasix)

   b. chlorothiazide (Diuril)

   c. spironolactone (Aldactone)

   d. mannitol (Osmitrol)

9. Your client is taking hydrochlorothiazide (HydroDIURIL) for ankle edema. On a follow-up visit to the clinic, she states that she has taken her medication as prescribed but continues to have swelling. You should assess for:

   a. alcohol intake

   b. sodium intake in her diet

   c. activity level

   d. possible drug–drug interactions

10. Your client has been on hydrochlorothiazide (HydroDIURIL) therapy for 3 weeks. Which of the following serum potassium levels indicate she is experiencing hypokalemia?

    a. 2.8 mEq/L

    b. 3.9 mEq/L

    c. 4.1 mEq/L

    d. 5 mEq/L

■Nephron Diagram

Fill in the blanks in Figure 44-1 with the terms below.

Descending limb of Henle's loop
Glomerulus
Ascending limb of Henle's loop
Henle's loop
Efferent arteriole

Bowman's capsule
Afferent arteriole
Distal tubule
Collecting tubule
Proximal tubule

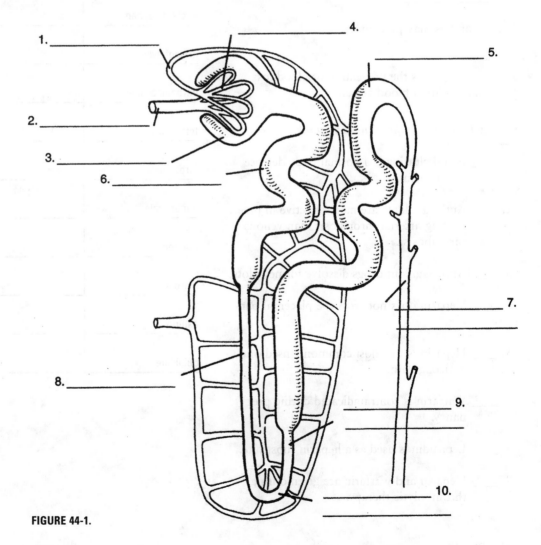

1. _____

2. _____

3. _____

4. _____

5. _____

6. _____

7. _____

8. _____

9. _____

10. _____

FIGURE 44-1.

CHAPTER 45

Drugs That Affect Blood Coagulation

■ Exercises

Fill in the blank.

1. _____ involves the formation or presence of a blood clot in a blood vessel.

2. An _____ is part of a thrombus that breaks off and travels to another part of the body.

3. Pathologic thrombosis is often the result of _____.

4. A thrombus may precipitate _____ _____.

5. _____ is the prevention of blood loss from an injured blood vessel.

Place a T (true) or F (false) in each blank.

1. ____ Blood clotting is a normal body defense mechanism.

2. ____ Anticoagulants are more effective in preventing arterial thrombosis than venous thrombosis.

3. ____ Anticoagulant drugs dissolve formed clots.

4. ____ Heparin does not cross the placental barrier.

5. ____ Heparin is the most commonly used oral anticoagulant.

6. ____ Warfarin is contraindicated during pregnancy.

7. ____ Lepirudin is used as a heparin substitute.

8. ____ Heparin and warfarin are given during thrombolytic therapy.

9. ____ Protamine sulfate is an antidote for heparin.

10. ____ Ginkgo can decrease the effects of warfarin.

Indicate whether the drug increases or decreases the effect of warfarin by placing a check in the appropriate column.

Drug	Increases	Decreases
acetaminophen		
griseofulvin		
carbamazepine		
tetracycline		
furosemide		
fluconazole		
rifampin		
estrogen		
aspirin		
quinidine		

■ Clinical Challenge

Your client is a 32-year-old nursing student who develops deep vein thrombosis (DVT) in her left leg. She is hospitalized, and an initial assessment reveals that she has been on birth control pills for 3 months. She is to receive IV heparin, 30 units/kg of body weight on admission and 20,000 units every 24 hours by IV infusion. Bedrest is ordered. Why is heparin the drug of choice for your client? Which laboratory tests will be ordered for her, and how often will it be done? Why will you monitor her response to the medication?

■ Review Questions

1. Your client is receiving intermittent IV doses of heparin. A nursing action related to heparin administration would be to:

   a. massage back and legs

   b. observe for signs and symptoms of hemorrhage

   c. ambulate client three times a day

   d. protect IV bag and tubing from the light

2. As a nurse, you would know to have which of the following drugs available when a client is on heparin therapy?

   a. vitamin K

   b. aminocaproic acid (Amicar)

   c. protamine sulfate

   d. tranexamic acid

3. Heparin is contraindicated in a client with:

   a. deep vein thrombosis

   b. cirrhosis

   c. peptic ulcer disease

   d. acute myocardial infarction

4. A client has started warfarin (Coumadin) therapy for deep vein thrombosis. She asks the nurse how long it will be before the drug starts breaking up the clots. The nurse's response should be:

   a. "I'm not sure, but I'll ask your doctor."

   b. "It will take about 3 to 5 days for the anticoagulant effects to occur."

   c. "We should be able to see positive results in 24 hours."

   d. "Anticoagulant effects will start immediately."

5. Your client is on continuous IV heparin therapy. What time should blood be drawn for the partial thromboplastin time?

   a. at any time

   b. 6 AM

   c. 12 noon

   d. 9 PM

6. Your client has intermittent claudication from peripheral vascular disease in both legs. She is taking cilostazol. Which of the following would be a desired outcome of drug therapy for her?

   a. decreased shortness of breath

   b. walking a quarter mile without leg pain

   c. decreased blood pressure

   d. participation in a 2-mile Heart Walk

7. A client is receiving warfarin (Coumadin). She should be scheduled for which of the following laboratory tests to monitor drug effectiveness?

   a. prothrombin time (PT) only

   b. international normalized ratio and PT

   c. activated partial thromboplastin time and PT

   d. international normalized ratio (INR) only

8. Your client is to receive heparin 5000 units SC. When administering this medication, you should:

   a. pull the skin tight with thumb and forefinger before injecting the medication

   b. aspirate the syringe for possible blood return

   c. massage the area for 1 minute once the medication is administered and the needle removed

   d. avoid aspirating the syringe and massaging the injection site

9. A client in the cardiac care unit is receiving an IV of streptokinase infusion for a suspected acute myocardial infarction. During the administration of this drug, the nurse will monitor the client for:

   a. headache

   b. skin rash

   c. dry mouth

   d. increased blood pressure

10. Your client is taking warfarin (Coumadin) for continued therapy for myocardial infarction. You observe that she has hematuria and gingival bleeding. You will plan to administer:

    a. vitamin K

    b. protamine sulfate

    c. aspirin

    d. alteplase

CHAPTER 46

Drugs for Dyslipidemia

■ Exercises

Fill in the blank.

1. Blood lipids include _____, _____, and _____.

2. Blood lipids are transported in plasma by _____.

3. _____ cholesterol is involved in the formation of atherosclerotic plaques.

4. _____ is used to reduce LDL cholesterol further in clients who are already receiving statin drugs.

5. The drug _____ is a statin, which can reduce low-density lipoprotein (LDL) cholesterol within 2 weeks.

6. _____ are useful for clients who have low high-density lipoprotein (HDL) cholesterol levels.

7. A _____ agent is recommended for single-drug therapy to lower cholesterol.

8. _____ is the preferred dyslipidemic for clients with diabetes mellitus.

9. _____ and _____ may cause hepatotoxicity.

10. _____ is a food source that is known to lower cholesterol.

Complete the chart.

Blood lipid	Desired level	Borderline level	High level
Triglycerides			
Total serum cholesterol			
LDL Cholesterol			
HDL Cholesterol			

Place a T (true) or F (false) in each blank.

1. ____ Drugs for dyslipidemia should be taken in the morning because more cholesterol is produced in the morning hours.

2. ____ Statin-type dyslipidemics may increase sensitivity to sunlight.

3. ____ Cholesterol is necessary for normal body functioning.

4. ____ HDL transports cholesterol away from arteries and back to the liver, where it is broken down.

5. ____ Type III dyslipidemia is characterized by lipid deposits in the feet, knees, and elbows.

6. ____ LDL cholesterol has protective effects against coronary heart disease.

7. ____ Fibrate agents may cause gallstones.

8. ____ Estrogen replacement therapy increases HDL cholesterol.

9. ____ Dyslipidemic drugs may be given to children younger than 10 years of age.

10. ____ Statins are contraindicated in clients with active liver disease.

▪ Clinical Challenge

Your client is 42 years old and is in the clinic for his annual physical. It is determined that his total serum cholesterol is 330 mg/dL. He becomes very upset and reveals that his father died when he was 48 years old from a "heart attack." The doctor decides to place him on niacin and asks you to discuss lifestyle changes with him. Discuss your teaching plans. What teaching will be needed regarding his medication?

▪ Review Questions

1. Which of the following clients receiving gemfibrozil (Lopid) needs special instruction?
   a. a 52-year-old male bus driver
   b. a 25-year-old housewife
   c. a 73-year-old retired female teacher
   d. a 42-year-old sales associate

2. A client who has hyperlipidemia and is taking lovastatin (Mevacor) should be instructed to take the medication:
   a. with the evening meal
   b. at 12 noon with lunch
   c. 2 hours after breakfast
   d. at 9 PM before bedtime

3. Your client has high cholesterol and triglycerides. Her health care provider has prescribed niacin (nicotinic acid). During a follow-up visit, she complains of skin flushing. An appropriate response to her would be:
   a. "This is an adverse effect that will continue as long as you take the medication."
   b. "Don't worry about it. It's really not that noticeable."
   c. "Take 325 mg of ASA 30 minutes prior to the niacin dose. This should decrease the flushing."
   d. "You need to stop the medication immediately. I will notify your physician."

4. Which of the following may be responsible for noncompliance with statin therapy in older adults?
   a. severe adverse effects
   b. cost of the medication
   c. bitter taste of the medication
   d. frequency of dosage

5. A client who is taking cholestyramine (Questran) will most likely experience which of the following adverse effects?
   a. headache
   b. rash
   c. diarrhea
   d. constipation

6. Which of the following drugs may decrease the
   effects of lovastatin (Mevacor)?
   a. antacids
   b. alcohol
   c. erythromycin
   d. niacin

7. A client is taking atorvastatin (Lipitor). Which
   of the following should **not** be ingested with the
   drug?
   a. sweet potatoes
   b. grapefruit juice
   c. peanuts
   d. canned tuna

8. Your client has been diagnosed with type IV
   dyslipidemia. Which of the following laboratory
   tests should be performed prior to and during
   therapy?
   a. creatinine clearance and specific gravity
   b. blood glucose level
   c. serum aspartate and alanine aminotransferase
   d. complete blood count

9. Fenofibrate (Tricor) is contraindicated in which
   of the following conditions?
   a. hepatotoxicity
   b. severe renal impairment
   c. diabetes mellitus
   d. peptic ulcer disease

10. Which of the following dyslipidemic agents is
    most effective for reducing serum triglyceride
    levels?
    a niacin (Nicotinic acid)
    b. gemfibrozil (Lopid)
    c. glycerin (Glycerol)
    d. triamterene (Dyrenium)

CHAPTER 47

Drugs Used for Peptic Ulcer and Acid Reflux Disorders

■ Exercises

Place a T (true) or F (false) in each blank.

1. ____ Gastric and duodenal ulcers are less common than esophageal ulcers.

2. ____ Pepsinogen is converted to pepsin when the pH of gastric juices is 3 or less.

3. ____ Smokers are more likely to develop duodenal ulcers.

4. ____ Gastroesophageal reflux disease (GERD) is common in people after 40 years of age.

5. ____ Antacids act primarily in the small intestine.

6. ____ Calcium compounds are used to treat peptic ulcer disease.

7. ____ Magnesium-based antacids are contraindicated in clients with renal failure.

8. ____ Cimetidine (Tagamet) is administered by the oral route only.

9. ____ Proton pump inhibitors are the drugs of first choice in most gastric and duodenal ulcers.

10. ____ Most cases of peptic ulcer disease are caused by a *Helicobacter pylori* infection.

Fill in the blank.

1. _____ ulcers most often are manifested by painless upper gastrointestinal bleeding.

2. _____ is a hormone released by cells in the stomach in response to food ingestion.

3. Commonly used antacids are _____, _____, and calcium compounds.

4. A _____ preparation exerts antibacterial effects against *H. pylori*.

5. _____ is more likely to cause mental confusion and gynecomastia than are other histamine-2 receptor antagonists.

6. _____, the first proton pump inhibitor, binds to the gastric proton pump to prevent the release of gastric acid.

7. _____ is used concurrently with nonsteroidal anti-inflammatory drugs (NSAIDs) to protect gastric mucosa from NSAID-induced erosion and ulceration.

8. A drug used in healing duodenal ulcers and in maintenance therapy to prevent the recurrence of ulcers is _____.

9. _____ increases blood level of diazepam.

10. _____ and _____ are contraindicated in clients with impaired renal function.

Match the following.

1. ____ pepsin

2. ____ gastric ulcers

3. ____ GERD

4. ____ proton pump inhibitors

5. ____ pyrosis

6. ____ gastritis

7. ____ gastropathy

8. ____ antacid

9. ____ *H. pylori*

10. ____ duodenal ulcers

a. Associated with stress, NSAID ingestion, and *H. pylori* infection; manifested by painless bleeding

b. Gram-negative bacterium found in the gastric mucosa

c. Strongest gastric acid suppressants

d. Proteolytic enzyme that helps digest protein foods

e. Acute gastritis resulting from irritation of the gastric mucosa

f. Caused by *H. pylori* infection and NSAID ingestion; associated with abdominal pain

g. An acute or chronic inflammatory reaction of gastric mucosa

h. Regurgitation of gastric content into the esophagus

i. Heartburn from gastroesophageal reflux disease (GERD)

j. An alkaline substance that neutralizes acids

■ Clinical Challenge

Your client is an 81-year-old male who was admitted to the hospital through the emergency department. He has been vomiting blood for the last 8 hours. Assessment data reveal that he has been taking prednisone, methotrexate, and Remicade for rheumatoid arthritis for the last 2 years. It is determined that he has a gastric ulcer. He is started on IV Protonix. After a weeklong stay in the hospital, the client is discharged and is to take Protonix PO. Why was Protonix ordered for this client? Identify adverse effects of Protonix. How

long do you suspect the client will have to take the medication? What instructions should be given to the client in regard to taking Protonix by mouth?

■ Review Questions

1. When teaching a client about taking antacids, the nurse will include which of the following information?

   a. Antacid tablets are not equal to the liquid form.

   b. Take antacids with food.

   c. Antacids absorb pepsin in the stomach.

   d. Do not take antacids with other medications.

2. Your client is taking sucralfate (Carafate). A potential nursing diagnosis for her would be:

   a. risk for constipation

   b. impaired urinary elimination

   c. activity intolerance

   d. deficient fluid volume

3. A 42-year-old male is being treated for a peptic ulcer with ranitidine (Zantac) 150 mg PO at bedtime. Even though few adverse effects have been associated with ranitidine, the nurse will inform the client of which of the following common adverse effects?

   a. headache

   b. irritability

   c. dry mouth

   d. fever

4. Your client is receiving drugs to prevent hyperacidity. An appropriate outcome for him would be:

   a. two formed stools per day

   b. loss of 2 pounds per week

   c. stools negative for occult blood

   d. increased appetite

5. Which of the following instructions would be given to a client in regard to administration of sucralfate (Carafate)?

   a. Take with meals.

   b. Take at least 1 hour before meals.

   c. Take after each meal.

   d. Take with a full glass of milk.

6. When evaluating a client on cimetidine therapy, which of the following laboratory tests should be performed?

   a. red blood cell count

   b. potassium level

   c. hepatic enzymes

   d. serum creatinine level

7. Your client is taking aluminum hydroxide. You expect the client to complain of:

   a. diarrhea

   b. constipation

   c. nausea

   d. headache

8. Your client is taking omeprazole (Prilosec). Which of the following is she being treated for?

   a. constipation

   b. GERD

   c. diarrhea

   d. asthma

9. A client has GERD and takes ranitidine (Zantac). She continues to have gastric discomfort and asks whether she can take an antacid. Your response should be:

   a. "Sure, you may take an antacid with Zantac."

   b. "No, the two drugs will be working against each other."

   c. "Yes, but be sure to wait at least 1 hour to take the antacid after you take the Zantac."

   d. "I wouldn't advise it. You may experience severe constipation."

10. Which of the following drugs would be indicated for a client who is taking NSAIDs for arthritis and is at high risk for gastrointestinal ulceration and bleeding?

    a. misoprostol (Cytotec)

    b. sucralfate (Carafate)

    c. lansoprazole (Prevacid)

    d. cimetidine (Tagamet)

CHAPTER 48

Antiemetics

■ Exercises

Fill in the blank.

1. The vomiting center is located in the _____ _____.

2. _____ and _____ are phenothiazines that are commonly used to prevent or treat nausea and vomiting.

3. _____ produce relaxation and inhibit the cerebral cortex input to the vomiting center.

4. _____ is a cannabinoid given to cancer patients to manage nausea and vomiting associated with chemotherapy.

5. _____ is used in the management of motion sickness.

6. An over-the-counter antiemetic given orally in 15-minute intervals is _____ _____.

7. _____ can be used as a transdermal patch to prevent seasickness.

8. _____ may increase the effects of alcohol and decrease the effects of digoxin.

9. The injectable form of _____ can be mixed in apple juice for clients who cannot swallow tablets.

10. A corticosteroid used in the management of chemotherapy-induced nausea and vomiting is _____.

Place a T (true) or F (false) in each blank.

1. ____ Antiemetics are more effective in preventing nausea and vomiting than in stopping them.

2. ____ Older adults are usually more sensitive to dronabinol's psychoactive effects than younger adults.

3. ____ Nausea must occur prior to vomiting.

4. ____ All antihistamines are effective as antiemetics.

5. ____ Benzodiazepines are considered antiemetics.

6. ____ Phenothiazines act on the CTZ and the vomiting center to exert antiemetic effects.

7. ____ Dronabinol (Marinol) has a high potential for abuse.

8. ____ Metoclopramide (Reglan) is contraindicated in Parkinson's disease.

9. ____ The 5-HT3 receptor antagonists are the first choice for clients with chemotherapy-induced nausea and vomiting.

10. ____ Large doses of phenothiazines are needed to produce antiemetic effects.

■ Clinical Challenge

Your client is a 55-year-old female who is receiving chemotherapy for colon cancer. She is experiencing nausea and vomiting related to her treatments. Ondansetron (Zofran) has been prescribed for her. Why was this drug ordered for the client? List common adverse effects of ondansetron (Zofran).

The client continues to complain of nausea and vomiting. Which drug do you suspect the physician will add to the client's antiemetic regimen?

▪ Review Questions

1. A 50-year-old is receiving promethazine (Phenergan) for chemotherapy-induced emesis. Because of anticholinergic effects, the nurse will encourage:
   a. frequent oral care
   b. increased fluid intake
   c. a low-fat diet
   d. ambulation

2. A client is receiving metoclopramide (Reglan) for severe nausea. The nurse will monitor the client for which of the following adverse effects?
   a. hypoglycemia
   b. dystonia
   c. GERD
   d. photosensitivity

3. Your client has been on antiemetic therapy. Which of the following statements indicate a need for further instruction?
   a. "I should avoid driving my car while taking my medication."
   b. "If I start losing weight, I should let you know."
   c. "I enjoy drinking a glass of red wine every night."
   d. "I have stopped going to my exercise class since I have been on medication."

4. Your client is taking dronabinol (Marinol) for nausea and vomiting associated with chemotherapy. A possible concern for the client when the drug is discontinued is:
   a. urinary frequency
   b. sleep disturbance
   c. joint pain and stiffness
   d. decreased appetite

5. Which of the following clients would **not** be a candidate for metoclopramide (Reglan) therapy?
   a. a 65-year-old male with congestive heart failure
   b. a 42-year-old female with breast cancer
   c. a 33-year-old female with diabetic gastroparesis
   d. a 50-year-old male with esophageal reflux

6. Which of the following antiemetic drugs should not be given to a child under the age of 12?
   a. promethazine (Phenergan)
   b. ondansetron (Zofran)
   c. dronabinol (Marinol)
   d. scopolamine (Transderm-Scop)

7. In older adults, a positive outcome of antiemetic therapy is:
   a. decrease in blood pressure
   b. weight gain of 2 pounds per week
   c. increased activity level
   d. electrolyte balance

8. Your client is taking an antiemetic. Which of the following nursing diagnoses would be appropriate for her?
   a. noncompliance: failure to take medication as prescribed
   b. injury: risk for
   c. disturbed sleep pattern
   d. inbalanced nutrition: more than body requirements

9. A 28-year-old female is in the clinic for antiemetic therapy. She is going on an ocean cruise and expects to experience motion sickness. Instructions regarding this medication will include:
   a. Take medication at first sign of nausea.
   b. Take 30 minutes prior to getting on the ship and then every 4 to 6 hours as needed.
   c. Take medication with food.
   d. Take 10 minutes before getting on the ship, then once a day throughout the cruise.

10. A client, age 40, is receiving chemotherapy for ovarian cancer. To decrease the adverse effects of the chemotherapy, the nurse will administer metoclopramide (Reglan):

    a. immediately after the chemotherapy treatment

    b. every 4 hours PO during the treatment

    c. IV 30 to 60 minutes prior to the chemotherapy treatment

    d. IM just prior to chemotherapy treatment

Answers

Chapter 1

DEFINITIONS

pharmacology—the study of drugs that alter functions of living organisms

biotechnology—involves manipulation of DNA and RNA in the development of drugs

drug therapy—the use of drugs to prevent, diagnose, or cure disease processes or to relieve signs and symptoms

prototypes—individual drugs that represent a group of drugs

medications—drugs that are given for therapeutic purposes

generic drug name—derived from the chemical or official name and is independent of a manufacturer

systemic drug effects—those resulting from drugs are absorbed into the bloodstream and circulated through the body

trade drug name—name given to a drug and patented by the manufacturer

synthetic chemical compounds—drugs manufactured in laboratories

over-the-counter (OTC)—refers to drugs that can be purchased without a prescription

SHORT ANSWER

1. Synthetic drugs are more standardized in chemical characteristics, more consistent in effects, and less likely to produce allergic reactions
2. Involves the costs of drug therapy, including purchasing, dispensing, storage, administration, laboratory, and other tests used to monitor client responses and losses from expiration
3. By prescription or order from licensed health care provider and by over-the-counter purchase of drugs that do not require a prescription
4. Trade names are capitalized; generic names are lowercase
5. According to their effects on certain body systems, their therapeutic uses, and chemical characteristics

FILL IN THE CHART

Name	Year	Provision
Comprehensive Drug Abuse Prevention and Control Act	1970	Regulated distribution of narcotics and other drugs of abuse
Durham-Humphrey	1952	Designated drugs that are prescribed by a physician and dispensed by a pharmacist
Kefauver-Harris Amendment	1962	Required proof that drugs were effective for how they were labeled
Harrison Narcotic Act	1914	Controlled the manufacture, importation, transportation, and distribution of opium, cocaine, marijuana, and their derivatives
Food, Drug and Cosmetic Act	1938	Regulated manufacture, distribution, advertising, and labeling of drugs

MATCHING

1. e 2. a 3. b 4. d 5. c 6. b 7. a 8. d
9. e 10. d

REVIEW QUESTIONS

1. b 2. a 3. c 4. c 5. b 6. c 7. b 8. c
9. d 10. a

Chapter 2

MATCHING

1. c 2. i 3. d 4. k 5. e 6. f 7. l 8. m
9. o 10. g 11. a 12. h 13. n 14. j 15. b

TRUE OR FALSE

1. f 2. t 3. f 4. t 5. f 6. t 7. t 8. f
9. t 10. f 11. t 12. f 13. t 14. t 15. t

DEFINITIONS

1. Involves drug movement from an area of higher concentration to one of lower concentration
2. Similar to passive diffusion except drug molecules combine with a carrier protein or enzyme
3. Drug molecules move from an area of lower concentration to one of higher concentration; requires a carrier substance and release of cellular energy

FILL IN THE CHART

Drug	Antidote
heparin	protamine sulfate
opioid analgesics	naloxone (Narcan)
phenothiazine	diphenhydramine (Benadryl)
warfarin (Coumadin)	vitamin K
acetaminophen	acetylcysteine (Mucomyst)
beta blockers	glucagon

REVIEW QUESTIONS

1. c   2. b   3. d   4. c   5. b   6. c   7. a   8. c
9. a   10. a

Chapter 3

FILL IN THE BLANK

1. metric
2. units
3. milliequivalents
4. decimal
5. household
6. Clark's rule
7. body surface area
8. drop factor
9. 60
10. apothecary and household

FILL IN THE BLANK: EQUIVALENT

1. 2.2   2. 1000   3. 1   4. 1   5. 15 or 16
6. 250   7. 1000   8. 1   9. 4 or 5   10. 1

FILL IN THE BLANK: CONVERSION

1. 30   2. 22.73   3. 8 or 10
4. 3.5   5. 10 or 12.5   6. 15
7. 2000   8. 2   9. 2
10. 2500

CALCULATING DRUG DOSAGES

1. 4 tablets
2. 10 mL
3. 60 mL
4. 1.5 mL
5. 2 tablets
6. 11.25 mL

7. 2 capsules
8. 0.5 mL
9. 2 mL
10. 15 cc

Chapter 4

DEFINITIONS

1. Right drug, dose, client, route, time, documentation, and right to refuse
2. The nurse is liable for his/her actions and is expected to have knowledge concerning all medications he/she is responsible for administering.
3. Name of client; generic or trade name of the drug; the dose, the route and frequency of administration; and the date, time, and signature of the prescriber
4. Any route other than gastrointestinal—denotes SC, IM, and IV
5. Because they contain high amounts of a drug intended to be absorbed slowly and act over an extended period of time; acts as an overdose

TRUE OR FALSE

1. f   2. t   3. t   4. f   5. f   6. t   7. t   8. t
9. f   10. f   11. t   12. f

MATCHING

1. g   2. m   3. j   4. e   5. o   6. i   7. b   8. c
9. d   10. f   11. a   12. k   13. l   14. h   15. n

REVIEW QUESTIONS

1. b   2. c   3. d   4. b   5. d   6. d   7. d   8. d
9. a   10. a

Chapter 5

FILL IN THE BLANK

1. nursing process
2. assessment
3. client
4. outcomes
5. clinical practice guidelines

SHORT ANSWER

1. Deficient knowledge: drug therapy regimen; deficient knowledge: safe and effective self-administration; risk for injury related to adverse drug effects; noncompliance: overuse; noncompliance: underuse
2. Take drugs as prescribed; experience relief of s/s; accurately self-administer a drug; report use of herbal and dietary supplements
3. Assessment, drug administration, teaching, solving problems related to drug therapy, promoting compliance with prescribed drug therapy and identifying barriers to compliance, identifying

resources for obtaining medication
4. Promoting healthy lifestyles, exercise, rest, sleep, handwashing, positioning, assisting with cough and deep breathing, ambulating, heat and cold
5. Because most medications are self administered and clients need information and assistance to use drugs safely and effectively.
6. Emphasis on outpatient treatments, short hospitalization period, client's reluctance to admit to noncompliance
7. What do you know about the drugs you are currently taking? What other drugs have you taken in the past? Have you ever had an allergic reaction to a drug before? Can you afford to take your medications? How do you feel about taking your prescribed drugs?
8. The 1994 Dietary Supplement Health and Education Act (DSHEA) defined a dietary supplement as "a vitamin, a mineral, an herb, or other botanical used to supplement the diet." Herbs can be labeled according to their possible effects on the body but are not used to diagnose, prevent, relieve, or cure diseases unless approved by the FDA.
9. Use of supplements may keep the client from seeking treatment from a health care provider when indicated, and the products may interact with prescription drugs to decrease therapeutic effects or increase adverse effects.
10. Child's weight, age, and level of growth and development

TRUE OR FALSE
1. f 2. t 3. f 4. t 5. t 6. f 7. t 8. f
9. t 10. t 11. t 12. f 13. t 14. f 15. f

MATCHING
1. e 2. m 3. l 4. f 5. j 6. h 7. b 8. g
9. b 10. a 11. d 12. i 13. c 14. c and k 15. k

CLINICAL CHALLENGE
Assess ability to manage drug therapy regimen; assess for risk for noncompliance. Teach the client to report s/s, the importance of taking medications as prescribed, and keeping follow-up appointments. Name, age, health problems, allergies. Questions concerning prescription medications: Do you take prescription medication? If yes, what are the name(s), dose(s), frequency, specific times and reason(s) for use? Do you take as prescribed? Does anyone else help you with your medications? What information or instructions were you given about the medications? Do you think the medication is working for you? Do you take over-the-counter medications? If yes, what are they and why do you take them? Do you take herbs or dietary supplements? Do you take social drugs (coffee, tea, cola, alcohol, tobacco, or illegal drugs)?

REVIEW QUESTIONS
1. d 2. d 3. b 4. b 5. b 6. a 7. c 8. d
9. b 10. b

Chapter 6

MATCHING
1. d 2. j 3. h 4. b 5. g 6. c 7. a 8. e
9. f 10. i

SHORT ANSWER
1. The signal from nociceptors in peripheral tissues must be transmitted to the spinal cord, then to the hypothalamus and cerebral cortex in the brain.
2. A system within the body to relieve pain.
3. Binds with narcotic receptor to relieve pain by inhibiting the release of substance P in central and peripheral nerves, decreasing the perception of pain sensation in the brain
4. Analgesia, drowsiness to sleep to unconsciousness, decreased mental and physical activity, respiratory depression, nausea and vomiting, and pupil constriction
5. Further depress respirations
6. Agonists—include morphine and morphine-like drugs; produce prototypical narcotic effects. Antagonists—antidote drugs that reverse the effects of narcotic agonists. However, the drugs can have agonistic activity at some receptors and antagonistic activity at other receptors.
7. Reverse or block analgesia, CNS respiratory depression, compete with narcotics at narcotic receptors
8. There is no upper limit to the dosage that can be given to clients who have developed tolerance to previous dosages.
9. Oral doses go through extensive metabolism on their first pass through the liver.
10. Aggressiveness, restlessness, body aches, insomnia, piloerection, nausea and vomiting, diarrhea, increased body temperature, increased respiratory rate and blood pressure, abdominal and muscle cramps, dehydration, and weight loss

TRUE OR FALSE
1. f 2. t 3. f 4. t 5. t 6. f 7. f 8. t
9. t 10. t

CLINICAL CHALLENGE
Acute pain—will subside, do not want to cause drug addiction, given before pain or at onset.

Chronic pain—goal is to make the client comfortable, not worried about addiction, given around the clock

REVIEW QUESTIONS
1. b 2. b 3. d 4. a 5. a 6. b 7. b 8. a
9. a 10. b

Chapter 7

MATCHING
1. i   2. c   3. e   4. d   5. f   6. g   7. h   8. j
9. a   10. b

TRUE OR FALSE
1. f   2. t   3. f   4. t   5. t   6. f   7. t   8. t
9. f   10. t

MATCHING
1. h   2. e   3. j   4. f   5. i   6. g   7. c   8. d
9. a   10. b

CLINICAL CHALLENGE
Salicylate poisoning–stop the drug or decrease the dosage

REVIEW QUESTIONS
1. a   2. b   3. c   4. d   5. d   6. b   7. b   8. d
9. b   10. b

Chapter 8

MATCHING
1. h   2. j   3. a   4. i   5. d   6. e   7. b   8. f
9. c   10. g

SHORT ANSWER
1. Does not cause drowsiness
2. Highly lipid-soluble, allows drugs to enter CNS and perform their actions. Drugs redistributed to peripheral tissues, then slowly eliminated
3. Severe respiratory disease, severe liver or kidney disease, hypersensitivity reactions, history of alcohol and other drug abuse
4. Buspirone lacks muscle relaxant and anticonvulsant effects, does not cause sedation or physical or psychological dependence, does not increase CNS depression of alcohol and other drugs, and is not a controlled substance
5. To relieve anxiety or sleeplessness without permitting sensory perception, responsiveness to the environment, or alertness to drop below safe levels

FILL IN THE BLANK
1. chlordiazepoxide
2. zolpidem
3. midazolam
4. buspirone
5. hydroxyzine
6. alprazolam
7. zaleplon
8. sertraline
9. lorazepam
10. temazepam

TRUE OR FALSE
1. t   2. f   3. f   4. t   5. t   6. f   7. t   8. t
9. t   10. t

CLINICAL CHALLENGE
Increased anxiety, psychomotor agitation, insomnia, irritability, headache, tremor, palpitations, and confusion. Gradual tapering of the dose by reducing the dose by 10% to 25% every 1 to 2 weeks over 4 to 6 weeks. Should be monitored for a few weeks for withdrawal symptoms.

REVIEW QUESTIONS
1. c   2. d   3. a   4. b   5. a   6. c   7. a   8. b
9. a   10. b

Chapter 9

TRUE OR FALSE
1. f   2. t   3. t   4. t   5. f   6. t   7. f   8. t
9. f   10. t

SHORT ANSWER
1. Agitation, behavioral disturbances, delusions, disorganized speech, hallucinations, insomnia, and paranoia
2. Lack of pleasure, motivation, a blunted affect, poor grooming and hygiene, poor social skills, poor speech, and social withdrawal
3. Typical—older, have more adverse effects, act mainly on positive symptoms of schizophrenia
   Atypical—newer, fewer adverse effects, act on both positive and negative symptoms of schizophrenia
4. Nausea, vomiting, and intractable hiccups
5. Causes agranulocytosis, a life-threatening blood disease, occurs in first 3 weeks of therapy

FILL IN THE BLANK
1. clozapine
2. dopamine
3. schizophrenia
4. haloperidol
5. pimozide
6. clozapine
7. promethazine
8. thioridazine
9. extrapyramidal effects
10. jaundice

CLINICAL CHALLENGE
Assess how long he has had diagnosis and drug therapy history for diagnosis.

Drug therapy compliance: why he does not take this medication and assess for reasons–cost, adverse effect, etc. Include positive outcome of medication therapy (fewer hospitalizations).

REVIEW QUESTIONS

1. b   2. a   3. c   4. d   5. d   6. a   7. c   8. b
9. c   10. a

Chapter 10

SHORT ANSWER

1. Depression thought to result from deficiency of norepinephrine and or serotonin. Thought that antidepressant drugs increase amounts of one or both of these in the CNS synapse.
2. Corticotropin-releasing factor increased in depression, which leads to increase in cortisol, which leads to decrease in cortisol receptors, which leads to depression. Also, abnormalities in secretion of thyroid and growth hormones can lead to depression.
3. Immune system; genetic factors; environmental factors
4. Tricyclics (TCAs); monoamine oxidase inhibitors (MAOIs); selective serotonin reuptake inhibitors (SSRIs)
5. Normalizes abnormal neurotransmission systems in the brain by altering the amounts of neurotransmitters and number of receptors
6. Aged cheese and meats; concentrated yeast extracts; sauerkraut; fava beans
7. Client's age; medical condition; history of drug response; drug adverse effects
8. Are effective and produce fewer and milder adverse effects
9. To prevent overdose—suicide
10. Occurs 1 to 4 hours after drug ingestion, causes nystagmus, tremors, restlessness, seizures, hypotension, dysrhythmias, myocardial depression

FILL IN THE BLANK

1. 2.5
2. bupropion
3. depression
4. hyperglycemia
5. bupropion/venlafaxine
6. receptors
7. MAOIs,
8. fluoxetine
9. lithium
10. St. John's wort

FILL IN THE CHART

TCAs—sedation, orthostatic hypotension, cardiac dysrhythmias, blurred vision, dry mouth, constipation, urinary retention, weight gain, sexual dysfunction

SSRIs—nausea, diarrhea, weight loss, sexual dysfunction, anxiety, nervousness, insomnia

MAOIs—severe hypertension, blurred vision, constipation, dizziness, dry mouth, hypotension, urinary retention, hypoglycemia

MATCHING

1. f   2. j   3. e   4. b   5. a   6. h   7. d   8. i
9. g   10. c

CLINICAL CHALLENGE

The client has bipolar disorder, which is characterized by mood swings from depression to manic behavior. Will probably be placed on Lithium. Therapeutic effects seen in 7 to 10 days.

REVIEW QUESTIONS

1. c   2. c   3. c   4. b   5. b   6. c   7. d   8. a
9. c   10. b

Chapter 11

MATCHING

1. g   2. j   3. i   4. b   5. h   6. e   7. a   8. f
9. d   10. c

FILL IN THE BLANK

1. epilepsy
2. fever
3. partial
4. generalized
5. clonic
6. tonic
7. absence
8. status epilepticus
9. CNS, GI tract
10. lorazepam
11. lamotrigine
12. levetiracetam
13. oxcarbazepine
14. topiramate
15. valproic acid
16. zonisamide
17. phenytoin
18. phenytoin
19. oxcarbazepine, carbamazepine
20. ethosuximide

CLINICAL CHALLENGE

Find out what times of the day he takes his medication. Is it every 12 hours and does he follow that schedule? How often does he have a carbamazepine level done? Has he been ill, had nausea and vomiting, diarrhea? Has he been worried, extremely upset, or stressed? Has he lost or gained weight?

REVIEW QUESTIONS

1. b   2. a   3. b   4. c   5. c   6. b   7. c   8. b
9. a   10. c

Chapter 12

MATCHING

1. h   2. e   3. g   4. a   5. b   6. c   7. f   8. d

TRUE OR FALSE

1. t   2. f   3. t   4. t   5. f   6. t   7. f   8. t
9. f   10. t

SHORT ANSWER

1. Destruction or degenerative changes in dopamine-producing nerve cells
2. Control symptoms, maintain functional ability in activities of daily living, minimize adverse drug effects, and slow disease progression
3. Better control of symptoms, reduced dosage of individual drugs
4. Increases the effects of the anticholinergic drug
5. Anorexia, nausea and vomiting, orthostatic hypotension, cardiac dysrhythmias, dyskinesia, CNS stimulation (restlessness, agitation, confusion, and delirium), abrupt swings in motor function

CLINICAL CHALLENGE

Dyskinesia eventually develops in most people who take levodopa. It is due to the duration of therapy. Decreasing the dosage may help. Tell her that some people prefer the dyskinesia to decreased dosage and parkinsonism symptoms returning.

REVIEW QUESTIONS

1. b   2. a   3. c   4. b   5. a   6. a   7. b   8. d
9. c   10. b

Chapter 13

SHORT ANSWER

1. Neurological and musculoskeletal disorders, muscle spasms and cramps, spinal cord injury, and multiple sclerosis
2. Cause CNS depression; use cautiously in clients with impaired renal function, hepatic or respiratory depression, and those who must be alert for daily function.
3. To relieve pain, muscle spasm, and spasticity without impairing the ability to perform self-care activities of daily living
4. Anticholinergic effects (eg, dry mouth, constipation, urinary retention, tachycardia), drowsiness and dizziness
5. Deficient knowledge: safe use of skeletal muscle relaxants (SMR); Risk of injury: sedation and dizziness related to SMR

FILL IN THE BLANK

1. dantrolene
2. carisoprodol
3. baclofen
4. cyclobenzaprine
5. metaxalone
6. methocarbamol and cyclobenzaprine
7. orphenadrine
8. cyclobenzaprine
9. metaxalone, tizanidine
10. dantrolene
11. baclofen
12. methocarbamol
13. methocarbamol
14. dantrolene
15. tizanidine

CLINICAL CHALLENGE

1. Risk for injury related to drowsiness and dizziness
2. Deficient knowledge: adverse effect of the drug
3. Potential for hepatotoxicity

REVIEW QUESTIONS

1. c   2. a   3. b   4. a   5. c   6. b   7. a   8. b
9. b   10. c

Chapter 14

DEFINITIONS

1. Self-administration of a drug for prolonged periods producing physical or psychological dependence
2. A craving for a drug with unsuccessful attempts to decrease its use; compulsive drug-seeking behavior
3. Feelings of satisfaction and pleasure from taking a drug
4. Physiologic adaptation to chronic use of a drug so that unpleasant symptoms occur when the drug is stopped
5. When the body adjusts to drugs so that higher doses are needed to achieve feelings of pleasure

SHORT ANSWER

1. Anxiety, tremors, muscle twitching, weakness, dizziness, distorted visual perceptions, N & V, insomnia, nightmares, tachycardia, weight loss, postural hypotension, tonic/clonic seizures, delirium, convulsions
2. Agitation, anxiety, tremors, sweating, nausea, tachycardia, fever, hyperreflexia, postural hypotension, convulsions, delirium
3. Sympathetic nervous system overactivity
4. Anxiety, irritability, difficulty concentrating, restlessness, headache, increased appetite, weight gain, sleep disturbances

TRUE OR FALSE

1. t   2. f   3. t   4. t   5. f   6. t   7. f   8. t
9. t   10. t

MATCHING

1. j   2. f   3. i   4. g   5. a   6. h   7. c   8. e
9. d   10. b

CLINICAL CHALLENGE

Convulsions and delirium will be in the first 72 hours.
Administration of benzodiazepine or phenobarbital to
relieve acute signs and symptoms. Will need to monitor
client for 72 hours.

REVIEW QUESTIONS

1. c   2. a   3. b   4. b   5. d   6. a   7. b   8. d
9. a   10. c

Chapter 15

FILL IN THE BLANK

1. narcolepsy
2. amphetamines
3. caffeine
4. Ritalin
5. modafinil
6. caffeine
7. No-Doz
8. doxapram
9. modafinil
10. theophylline

SHORT ANSWER

Chapter 16

FILL IN THE CHART

Espresso—120 mg
Iced tea—70 mg
Mr. Pibb—57 mg
Mountain Dew—54 mg
Instant tea—50 mg
Coke—45 mg
Diet Pepsi—38 mg

FILL IN THE CHART

Drug	Narcolepsy	ADHD
Amphetamine	x	x
Dexedrine	x	x
Provigil	x	
Adderall	x	x
Desoxyn		x
Focalin		x
Ritalin	x	x

CLINICAL CHALLENGE

Falling asleep in court could be embarrassing for this
client and could affect a legal outcome. Modafinil
(Provigil) might be prescribed. The outcome of this drug is
to promote wakefulness.

REVIEW QUESTIONS

1. a   2. d   3. b   4. c   5. a   6. d   7. a   8. b
9. a   10. c

FILL IN THE CHART

Alpha and beta activity	Alpha activity	Beta activity
dopamine (Intropin)	metaraminol (Aramine)	albuterol (Proventil)
epinephrine (Adrenalin)	oxymetazoline hydrochloride (Afrin)	terbutaline (Brethine)
ephedrine (Efedron)	phenylephrine (Neo-Synephrine)	isoproterenol (Isuprel)
norepinephrine (Levophed)	tetrahydrozoline hydrochloride (Visine)	dobutamine (Dobutrex)
pseudoephedrine (Sudafed)	tuaminoheptane (Tuamine)	isoetharine (Bronkosol)

MATCHING

1. e   2. g   3. g   4. e   5. j and c   6. e, f, and g
7. g   8. c and j   9. e   10. a and e

TRUE OR FALSE

1. t   2. t   3. f   4. f   5. t   6. f   7. t   8. f
9. t   10. t

CLINICAL CHALLENGE

Administer between 0.1 and 0.5 mg in a tuberculin
syringe. Massage injection site to increase absorption.
Client should expect relief in about 5 minutes.

REVIEW QUESTIONS

1. a   2. c   3. b   4. c   5. c   6. d   7. b   8. b
9. c   10. c

Chapter 17

SHORT ANSWER

1. Decreases urinary retention and improves urine flow by inhibiting contraction of muscle in the prostate and urinary bladder
2. Decrease in heart rate, cardiac output, blood pressure, and aqueous humor in the eye, and bronchoconstriction
3. To suppress pathologic stimulation, not the normal physiologic response to activity, stress, and other stimuli
4. Drugs combine with alpha-1 and beta-1 and -2 in peripheral tissues and prevent adrenergic effects
5. Inhibits release of norepinephrine in the brain, decreasing effects of sympathetic nervous system, which leads to a decrease in blood pressure

MATCHING

1. f 2. c 3. h 4. g 5. i 6. a 7. j 8. e
9. d 10. b

FILL IN THE CHART

Drug	Angina	Myocardial infarction	Tachydysrhythmia	Hypertension	Glaucoma
atenolol	x	x			
metoprolol	x	x			
nadolol	x				
propranolol	x	x	x	x	
acebutolol			x		
esmolol			x		
sotalol			x		
timolol		x		x	x
betaxolol				x	x
carteolol				x	x
levobunolol					x
metipranolol					x

CLINICAL CHALLENGE

Propranolol relieves palpitations and angina and decreases heart rate. The drug will be taken once or twice daily. The client should not discontinue drug abruptly. Blood pressure and pulse rate should be checked frequently. Adverse effects may include decreased pulse, bronchospasms, dyspnea, wheezing, fatigue, dizziness (especially with activity or exercise), depression, insomnia, vivid dreams and hallucinations. Antacids can decrease the effects of propranolol. Report weight gain of more than 2 pounds a week, ankle edema, shortness of breath, or extreme fatigue. Consult MD if taking over-the-counter drugs. The duration of drug therapy will depend on the client's response and cessation of symptoms.

REVIEW QUESTIONS

1. b 2. b 3. a 4. c 5. a 6. d 7. b 8. a
9. c 10. a

DIAGRAM

1. Epinephrine and norepinephrine
2. Beta adrenergic blocking drug
3. Nerve ending
4. Receptor site on cell surface
5. Myocardial or other tissue cell

Chapter 18

FILL IN THE BLANK

1. parasympathetic
2. nicotinic
3. glaucoma
4. bethanechol
5. tacrine, donepezil, rivastigmine
6. neostigmine
7. edrophonium

8. physostigmine salicylate
9. pyridostigmine
10. donepezil
11. rivastigmine
12. tacrine
13. pyridostigmine
14. physostigmine
15. atropine

TRUE OR FALSE

1. t 2. f 3. t 4. f 5. t 6. f 7. t 8. t
9. f 10. t

CLINICAL CHALLENGE

Increased muscle weakness, difficulty breathing, or recurrence of myasthenic symptoms are signs of drug underdosage (myasthenic crisis) and indicate a need to increase or change drug therapy. Positive outcome of drug therapy would be decreased or absent ptosis of eyelids; decreased difficulty with chewing, swallowing, and speech; increased skeletal strength; increased tolerance of activity; and less fatigue.

REVIEW QUESTIONS

1. b 2. d 3. d 4. c 5. c 6. a 7. d 8. b
9. b 10. c

Chapter 19

MATCHING

1. d 2. a 3. g 4. h 5. f 6. e 7. c 8. b
9. i 10. j

SHORT ANSWER

1. Blocks the action of acetylcholine on the parasympathetic nervous system.
2. Stimulation followed by depression of the CNS; decreased cardiovascular response; bronchodilation, and decreased respiratory tract secretions; antispasmodic effects in gastrointestinal tract (decreased muscle tone and motility); and mydriasis in the eye
3. To prevent vagal stimulation and potential bradycardia, hypotension, and cardiac arrest
4. To decrease the spasm-producing effects of the opioid analgesic
5. Hyperthermia-hot, dry, flushed skin; dry mouth; mydriasis; delirium; tachycardia; ileus and urinary retention
6. Tertiary amines-excreted in urine, lipid soluble, well absorbed from GI tract, crosses blood brain barrier quaternary amines-excreted in feces, lipid insoluble, poorly absorbed from GI tract and does not cross the blood brain barrier
7. Causes secretions to thicken and form mucus plugs in airways

8. Have been associated with behavioral disturbances and psychotic reactions
9. Blurred vision, confusion, heat stroke, constipation, urinary retention, hallucinations
10. Dilation of blood vessels in the neck

CLINICAL CHALLENGE

Dx: Constipation related to slowed gastrointestinal function
Goal: The client will defecate daily

Dx: Deficient knowledge: adverse effects of drug
Goal: The client will understand adverse effects of anticholinergic drug therapy

Dx: Disturbed thought processes: confusion and disorientation
Goal: The client will be oriented to person, place, and time

REVIEW QUESTIONS

1. c 2. a 3. b 4. a 5. c 6. d 7. a 8. b
9. c 10. d

Chapter 20

MATCHING

1. h 2. d 3. e 4. k 5. i 6. f 7. a 8. m
9. c 10. g 11. b 12. o 13. n 14. j 15. l

TRUE OR FALSE

1. f 2. f 3. t 4. t 5. t 6. f 7. f 8. t
9. t 10. f

CLINICAL CHALLENGE

To help slow bone loss and to help prevent loss of height, back pain, and spinal deformity or fracture.

Corticosteroids, phenytoin, alcohol and caffeine.

Take with 6 to 8 oz of water at least 30 minutes before ingesting any food, fluids, or other medication because other fluids and foods can decrease absorption and effectiveness. Take in upright position. Do not lie down for at least 30 minutes. This helps prevent stomach upset and irritation of the esophagus.

REVIEW QUESTIONS

1. a 2. b 3. a 4. b 5. b 6. d 7. b 8. c
9. c 10. b

Chapter 21

FILL IN THE BLANK

1. iodine, tyrosine
2. simple goiter
3. levothyroxine
4. protein

5. levothyroxine
6. thioamide
7. iodine
8. liothyronine
9. TSH
10. intracellular protein synthesis

MATCHING

1. f   2. j   3. a   4. d   5. h   6. i   7. g   8. c
9. e   10. b

TRUE OR FALSE

1. f   2. t   3. t   4. f   5. t   6. f   7. f   8. t
9. f   10. t

CLINICAL CHALLENGE

Find out why she thinks her dose may have to be increased. It is possible that symptoms of hypothyroidism may still be present. Tell her to take medication on an empty stomach because it increases absorption of the drug. Stress that this will be lifelong therapy. Periodic serum TSH levels will be needed; monitor blood pressure and pulse; don't take if the pulse is over 100; monitor weight; get adequate amounts of fluid. Encourage activity; skin care is important. Avoid ephedra. Take on an empty stomach and do not take with antacid.

REVIEW QUESTIONS

1. a   2. a   3. c   4. c   5. c   6. c   7. a   8. b
9. d   10. a

Chapter 22

MATCHING

1. e   2. c   3. d   4. g   5. h   6. j   7. i   8. f
9. a   10. b

TRUE OR FALSE

1. t   2. f   3. t   4. f   5. f   6. t   7. t   8. f
9. t   10. t   11. f   12. t   13. f   14. f   15. f   16. f
17. t   18. t   19. f   20. t

FILL IN THE CHART

Type	Onset	Peak	Duration
Regular Iletin II	½–1 hour	2–3 hours	5–7 hours
NPH	1–1½ hours	8–12 hours	18–24 hours
Humalog	15 minutes	½–1½ hours	6–8 hours
Humulin N	1–1½ hours	8–12 hours	18–24 hours
Ultralente	4–8 hours	10–30 hours	36 hours
Novolin R	½–1 hour	2–3 hours	5–7 hours

CLINICAL CHALLENGE

Metformin (Glucophage) will most likely be ordered. Age, type of diabetes, allergy to sulfa drugs. Does not cause weight gain. Assessment of hepatic and renal function and cardiac and respiratory function.

REVIEW QUESTIONS

1. c   2. a   3. b   4. d   5. b   6. d   7. b   8. d
9. b   10. a

Chapter 23

TRUE OR FALSE

1. f   2. f   3. t   4. t   5. f   6. t   7. t   8. f
9. t   10. f   11. t   12. t   13. f   14. f   15. t

MATCHING

1. a   2. d   3. c   4. b   5. i   6. e   7. j   8. h
9. f   10. g

CLINICAL CHALLENGE

0.1 mg/minute initially—will increase by 50 mcg/minute every 10 minutes to a maximal dose of 350 mcg/minute Should be continued for 12 hours after uterine contractions stop.

On her left side.

Ritodrine can cause hyperglycemia. Insulin dosage may need to be increased. Will have to be monitored very carefully. Other adverse effects include heart palpitations, dysrhythmias, changes in blood pressure, nausea and vomiting; dyspnea and chest pain may occur.

REVIEW QUESTIONS

1. b   2. c   3. b   4. b   5. b   6. c   7. d   8. b
9. a   10. d

Chapter 24

TRUE OR FALSE

1. t   2. t   3. f   4. f   5. f   6. t   7. t   8. t
9. f   10. f

SHORT ANSWER

1. Promotes growth in tissues related to reproduction and sexual characteristics
2. To prevent endometrial cancer
3. Pregnancy, thromboembolic disorders, suspected breast or genital tissues cancer, undiagnosed vaginal or uterine bleeding, fibroid tumors of the uterus, stroke victims, heart disease, family history of breast cancer
4. Inhibits hypothalamic secretion of gonadotropin-releasing hormone, which inhibits pituitary secretion of FSH and LH, which stops ovulation; produces mucus that resists penetration of sperm into upper reproductive tract; interferes with endometrial maturation and reception of ova that are released and fertilized

FILL IN THE BLANK

1. progesterone
2. liver
3. estrogen
4. progesterone
5. ethinyl estradiol
6. black cohosh
7. Preven
8. Estraderm
9. gonadorelin (Lutrepulse)
10. bromocriptine (Parlodel)

CLINICAL CHALLENGE

Assess for hysterectomy, intact uterus and ovaries, factors that may precipitate the fatigue and hot flashes; her knowledge concerning treatment of menopause. It will be important to keep annual checkups with her health care provider, have yearly mammograms and cardiac workups. Diet and weight should be discussed. Should increase calcium intake. Watch for vaginal bleeding. Encourage her to evaluate her need for hormone replacement therapy in 2 years and possibly consider coming off the hormones.

REVIEW QUESTIONS

1. c   2. b   3. d   4. a   5. a   6. d   7. b   8. b
9. d   10. b

Chapter 25

SHORT ANSWER

1. Testes, ovaries, and adrenal cortices
2. Development of male sexual characteristics; reproduction; and metabolism
3. Because of abuse potential
4. Hypertension, decreased HDL, increased LDL, benign and malignant neoplasms, aggression, hostility, combativeness, decreased testicular function, amenorrhea, acne

FILL IN THE BLANK

1. cholesterol
2. estrogens
3. testosterone
4. Testoderm
5. scrotum
6. danazol
7. danazol
8. liver
9. Leydig's
10. proteins

CLINICAL CHALLENGE

"I'd be very worried if the rumor is true because anabolic steroids are abused, and nonprescription sales are illegal. However, they are easily obtained. They can stop bone growth and damage heart, kidneys and the liver. Cardiac disorders, reproductive disorders and changes in behavior can occur."

REVIEW QUESTIONS

1. b   2. b   3. b   4. b   5. a   6. d   7. a   8. d
9. d   10. c

Chapter 26

MATCHING

1. e   2. i   3. d   4. a   5. h   6. j   7. c   8. b
9. f   10. g

TRUE OR FALSE

1. t   2. f   3. f   4. t   5. t   6. t   7. t   8. f
9. f   10. f

CLINICAL CHALLENGE

The client will receive parenteral feeding to restore nutritional status and increase weight. Possibly for several weeks, and she will probably continue the feedings at home.

Encourage the client to eat as much as she can – small, frequent feedings. Talk about food preferences and her knowledge of nutrition. Promote increasing activity and monitor weight and intake and output.

REVIEW QUESTIONS

1. b   2. c   3. c   4. a   5. a   6. c   7. a   8. c
9. b   10. b

Chapter 27

MATCHING

1. h   2. f   3. b   4. j   5. e   6. d   7. g   8. i
9. c   10. a

TRUE OR FALSE

1. t   2. t   3. f   4. f   5. t   6. f   7. t   8. t
9. t   10. f

CLINICAL CHALLENGE

Tell her that none of the available weight loss drugs are indicated for use in children.

Teaching plan should include assessment of activity and diet. Encourage more active life style, low fat diet, more regular meals, no snacking, drinking water instead of calorie containing drinks, decrease time watching TV, participate in household chores.

REVIEW QUESTIONS

1. b   2. a   3. c   4. b   5. a   6. b   7. c   8. c
9. d   10. a

Chapter 28

MATCHING

1. j   2. a   3. i   4. d   5. g   6. b   7. h   8. c
9. f   10. e

FILL IN THE CHART

Bacteria pathogen	Gram-positive or gram-negative	Normal in body flora	Medical conditions
Escherichia coli	gram-negative	intestinal tract	urinary tract infection (UTI), pneumonia, sepsis
Enterococci	gram-positive	human intestines	nosocomial infections, endocarditis
Staphylococcus spp.	gram-positive	skin, upper respiratory tract	boils, carbuncles, burn and surgical wounds, abscesses
Bacteroides spp.	gram-negative	digestive, respiratory, genital tracts	intra-abdominal and pelvic abscesses, brain abscess, bacteremia
Klebsiella spp.	gram-negative	bowels, respiratory tract, urinary tract, burns, wounds, meninges, bloodstream	pneumonia, sepsis, bacteremia
Streptococcus spp.	gram-positive	throat and nasopharynx	UTI, pneumonia, sinusitis, otitis media, meningitis

SHORT ANSWER

1. Intact skin and mucous membranes, anti-infective secretions, mechanical movements, phagocytic cells, immune and inflammatory processes
2. Widespread use of antimicrobials, interrupted or inadequate treatment, type of bacteria, type of infection, condition of host, location or setting
3. Inhibition of bacterial wall synthesis, inhibition of protein synthesis, disruption of microbial cell membranes, inhibition of organism reproduction by interfering with nucleic acid, inhibition of cell metabolism and growth

REVIEW QUESTIONS

1. b   2. a   3. c   4. d   5. c   6. c   7. d   8. c
9. c   10. b

Chapter 29

SHORT ANSWER

1. Penicillins, cephalosporins, carbapenems, monobactams
2. Inhibit synthesis of bacterial cell walls by binding to proteins that produce defective cell walls, which causes intracellular contents to leak, destroying microorganisms
3. Protects the penicillin from destruction by the enzymes and extends the penicillin's antimicrobial activity
4. Because the drugs are chemically similar

MATCHING

1. j   2. g   3. h   4. b   5. i   6. d   7. e   8. f
9. c   10. a

TRUE OR FALSE

1. t   2. f   3. f   4. t   5. f   6. t   7. t   8. t
9. f   10. f

CLINICAL CHALLENGE

Take the entire prescription, even if he feels good. Space evenly over the 24 – hour period, before school, at 3:30 pm and before bedtime. Report any rash. Should be taken on empty stomach with full glass of water, no orange juice or acidic juices.

REVIEW QUESTIONS

1. c   2. a   3. b   4. d   5. a   6. b   7. b   8. a
9. d   10. b

Chapter 30

MATCHING

1. e   2. j   3. b   4. g   5. f   6. i   7. h   8. d
9. c   10. a

TRUE OR FALSE

1. f   2. t   3. t   4. t   5. f   6. f   7. t   8. f
9. t   10. t

CLINICAL CHALLENGE

Assess for impaired renal and liver function, inadequate fluid intake, frequent or prolonged exposure to sunlight, CBC. Avoid sun exposure and encourage fluids.

Pseudomembranous colitis

To stop taking the drug and that you will consult with her physician. This is common with this drug and is caused by

bacteria (*C. difficile*) that produce a toxin that kills mucosal cells and produces superficial ulcerations. Metronidazole therapy will be started.

REVIEW QUESTIONS

1. b 2. d 3. c 4. a 5. b 6. a 7. a 8. b 9. a 10. a

Chapter 31

SHORT ANSWER

1. Uncomplicated urethral, endocervical or rectal infections; adjunctive therapy for pelvic inflammatory disease (PID) and STDs; long-term acne; substitution for penicillin; traveler's diarrhea; inhibit antidiuretic hormone
2. Inhibits microlial protein synthesis
3. Act as antimetabolites of para-aminobenzoic acid (PABA) required to produce folic acid. Causes formation of nonfunctional derivatives of folic acid. Halts multiplication of new bacteria but does not kill mature, fully formed bacteria.
4. Deposited in bones and teeth along with calcium. Can cause permanent brown coloring of tooth enamel. Can cause fatal hepatic necrosis in the mother.

TRUE OR FALSE

1. f   2. t   3. t   4. f   5. t   6. f   7. f   8. t
9. t   10. t

CLINICAL CHALLENGE

Call attention to the fact that the client has indicated that he is allergic to sulfonamides.

REVIEW QUESTIONS

1. d   2. d   3. a   4. b   5. a   6. b
7. b   8. c   9. b   10. c

Chapter 32

SHORT ANSWER

1. Penetrates body cells and mycobacteria, kills actively growing intracellular and extracellular organisms, and inhibits growth of dormant organisms in macrophages and tuberculous lesions.
2. LTBI-mycobacteria is inactive but remains alive in the body. There are no symptoms and the infection does not spread to others. Will have a positive TB skin test. Can develop active TB later. Active-usually results from reactivation of latent infection. Will have persistent cough and productive sputum, chest pain, chill, fever, hemoptysis, night sweats, weight loss, weakness, lack of appetite. Will have positive skin test and abnormal chest x-ray.
3. An increase in drug-resistant infections.
4. By performing and reading TB skin tests, tracking

contacts, assessing clients/homes, etc., educating clients and families, administering prescribed drugs, and maintaining records.

5. Isoniazid, rifampin, pyrazinamide, ethambutol, and streptomycin

MATCHING

1. c 2. d 3. h 4. g 5. f 6. i 7. j 8. b 9. a 10. e

TRUE OR FALSE

1. t 2. t 3. t 4. f 5. f 6. t 7. t 8. t 9. f 10. t

CLINICAL CHALLENGE

Considered a follow-up visit, assess client's condition in relation to drug therapy, disease, etc. Assess for education needs with the family and the possibility of the spread of TB within the family and neighborhood.

COMPLETE THE CHART

Drug	Parasitic Infection
mebendazole (Vermox)	hookworms, pinworms, roundworms and whipworms
pyrantel (Antiminth)	roundworms, pinworms and hookworms
thiabendazole (Mintezol)	threadworms and pinworms
permethrin (Elimite)	pediculosis and scabies
malathion (Ovide)	pediculosis

CLINICAL CHALLENGE

Help her work through and accept diagnosis. She must be able to concentrate to understand drug therapy. Anemia may occur with two to four weeks of starting zidovudine. Have CBC done every 2 weeks. May experience peripheral numbness, debilitation, and fatigue.

Fever, chills, tachypnea, nephrotoxicity, hypokalemia

Report symptoms to physician immediately.

The medication should be taken PO (by mouth) one tablet weekly for two weeks before entering Africa, then eight weeks after leaving the area. Should be taken on the same day of the week each week and at approximately the same time. Acute symptoms are headache, malaise, fever, and chills. Wear long sleeves and long pants, sleep in screened areas. Mosquitoes are most active at dusk and dawn.

REVIEW QUESTIONS

1. b 2. b 3. a 4. d 5. b 6. c 7. a 8. a 9. a 10. a

1. a 2. a 3. d 4. b 5. c 6. b 7. d 8. b 9. a 10. d

Chapter 33

MATCHING

1. c 2. m 3. q 4. d 5. t 6. g 7. h 8. i 9. j 10. e 11. a 12. s 13. n 14. p 15. o 16. r 17. b 18. k 19. l 20. f

TRUE OR FALSE

1. t 2. f 3. f 4. t 5. t 6. f 7. t 8. t 9. f 10. t

Chapter 34

TRUE OR FALSE

1. t 2. f 3. t 4. f 5. f 6. f 7. f 8. t 9. t 10. f 11. t 12. f 13. t 14. t 15. t 16. t 17. f 18. f 19. t 20. t 21. t 22. t 23. t 24. f 25. t

CLINICAL CHALLENGE

Try to determine where her son received the vaccines as best she can and call for the records. May need to repeat some immunizations if records cannot be found. Stress the importance of keeping the record in a safe place and that immunizations help prevent disease.

REVIEW QUESTIONS

1. c 2. b 3. a 4. a 5. d 6. d 7. a 8. d 9. b 10. c

Chapter 35

SHORT ANSWER

1. To restore normal function or increase the ability of the immune system to eliminate harmful invaders
2. Difficulty in maintaining effective dose levels over treatment periods of weeks or months; some of the drugs have a short half-life and require frequent administration; are very powerful and cause adverse effects
3. Produce enzymes that inhibit protein synthesis and degrade viral RNA
4. Stimulates the immune system and elicits a local inflammatory response
5. They are proteins that would be destroyed by digestive enzymes.

FILL IN THE BLANK

1. oprelvekin
2. interferons
3. darbepoetin alfa, epoetin
4. aldesleukin
5. filgrastim
6. interferon alfa-2b
7. Avonex
8. antineoplastic
9. corticosteroids
10. interferons

CLINICAL CHALLENGE

It will make a difference in benefits and decrease adverse effects.

Keep in the refrigerator, do not shake, do not change brands, take at bedtime to decrease common adverse effects, take acetaminophen to prevent or decrease fever or headache.

Maintain good fluid intake – 2 to 3 quarts daily.

REVIEW QUESTIONS

1. d   2. d   3. b   4. d   5. b   6. d   7. c   8. a
9. b   10. a

Chapter 36

MATCHING

1. f   2. a   3. d   4. h   5. j   6. g   7. i   8. c
9. e   10. b

TRUE OR FALSE

1. t   2. f   3. t   4. f   5. t   6. t   7. f   8. t
9. f   10. t

CLINICAL CHALLENGE

Replacement of glucocorticoids and mineralocorticoids will be needed. Daily administration will be required and should be taken between 6 and 9 am. The goal is to decrease the symptoms of Addison's disease to a tolerable level. Drugs may increase blood sugar level and increase blood pressure. May need to increase medication during stressful situations. Drug will be for life. Encourage walking and staying active, eating a balanced diet, and reporting any infections. Take meds as prescribed and may take with meals. Will have to be monitored for diabetes, tuberculosis and peptic ulcer disease. Corticosteroids are used to treat cancer. The drugs should be beneficial in several s/s of cancer. They have strong antiemetic effects.

Determine what adverse effects he may be experiencing. Consult the physician if needed. Discuss side effects of all four drugs. Review signs and symptoms of infection, gastrointestinal upset, respiratory distress, hepatic toxicity and anemia. Determine which he is experiencing. Discuss alternative drugs that he might be able to take.

REVIEW QUESTIONS

1. c   2. b   3. c   4. c   5. a   6. a   7. a   8. b
9. a   10. d

Chapter 37

TRUE OR FALSE

1. f   2. t   3. t   4. f   5. t   6. f   7. t   8. f
9. f   10. f

FILL IN THE BLANK

1. formoterol, salmeterol
2. metaproterenol
3. terbutaline
4. ipratropium
5. theophylline
6. leukotrienes
7. zileuton
8. cromolyn and nedocromil
9. terbutaline
10. corticosteroid

CLINICAL CHALLENGE

Assessment—how soon does she use the inhaler after an attack begins? How severe are the attacks? Does she know what triggers the attacks? Ask her to demonstrate use of the inhaler.

Tell her to shake well. Exhale to end of normal breath with the inhaler in the upright position. Place the mouthpiece inside mouth and use lips to form tight seal. While pressing down on the inhaler, take slow, deep breaths for 3 to 5 minutes before taking second inhalation. Ask her physician about a spacer device and explain that it has a tube attached to the inhaler to make it easy to use.

REVIEW QUESTIONS

1. c 2. d 3. c 4. a 5. d 6. d 7. b 8. b
9. d 10. a

Chapter 38

SHORT ANSWER

1. Secretory granules of mast and basophils cells-mostly tissue of skin and mucosal surfaces of eye, nose, lungs, and GI tract
2. Response to certain stimuli (allergic reactions, cellular injury, and extreme cold)
3. Mainly on smooth muscle cells in blood vessels and the respiratory and GI tract
4. Contraction of smooth muscle in bronchi and bronchioles; stimulation of vagus nerve endings to produce reflex bronchoconstriction and cough; increase in permeability of veins and capillaries, which causes fluid to flow into subcutaneous tissues and form edema; increased secretions of mucous glands; stimulation of sensory peripheral nerve endings to cause pain and pruritus; dilation of capillaries in the skin to cause flushing
5. Increased secretion of gastric acid and pepsin; increased rate and force of myocardial contraction; decreased immunologic and inflammatory reactions

MATCHING

1. j 2. c 3. b 4. d 5. f 6. g 7. h 8. e
9. i 10. a

CLINICAL CHALLENGE

Does she drive, are there stairs in her home, does she live alone? Does she operate electrical appliances or any type of machinery? What kind of job does she have? Does she have rugs, clutter, etc. in the home?

REVIEW QUESTIONS

1. c 2. a 3. c 4. a 5. b 6. b 7. a 8. d
9. b 10. a

Chapter 39

DEFINITIONS

1. When the heart cannot pump enough blood to meet tissue needs for oxygen
2. A neurohormone that acts as a vasoconstrictor and may exert toxic effects on the heart, resulting in myocardial cell proliferation

3. Administration of a sufficient amount of digitalis to produce therapeutic effects

TRUE OR FALSE

1. t 2. t 3. f 4. t 5. t 6. f 7. f 8. t
9. t 10. f 11. t 12. f 13. f 14. f 15. t

MATCHING

1. e 2. g 3. c 4. h 5. d 6. i 7. j 8. a
9. b 10. f

CLINICAL CHALLENGE

Digoxin level, acid base, and electrolyte values will be monitored. Therapeutic range is 0.5 to 2.0 ng/mL.

Monitor her pulse rate daily and report it if it is below 60 beats per minute. Mare sure dose is accurate. Report response to drug to health care provider. Adverse effects include anorexia, nausea and vomiting, headache, drowsiness, confusion and visual disturbances.

Digoxin toxicity can occur with any drug serum level; consistent monitoring is extremely important. Explain that digoxin has a low therapeutic index. A dose adequate for therapeutic effects may decrease the heart rate greatly.

REVIEW QUESTIONS

1. b 2. a 3. a 4. c 5. c 6. a 7. b 8. b
9. b 10. a

Chapter 40

FILL IN THE BLANK

1. sodium, calcium, potassium
2. excitability
3. absolute refractory
4. relative refractory
5. conductivity
6. disturbances
7. hypomagnesemia
8. atrial fibrillation
9. digoxin
10. supraventricular tachydysrhythmias

MATCHING

1. j 2. i 3. b 4. c 5. e 6. d 7. g 8. a
9. f 10. h

CARDIAC ELECTROPHYSIOLOGY DIAGRAM

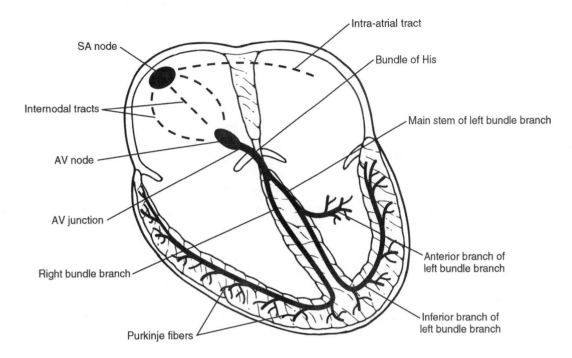

CLINICAL CHALLENGE
1 to 2 mg/kg.

Over a two minute period.

0 to 4 mg/min.

Digoxin levels should be in the 2 to 5 mcg/mL range. The nurse must be aware of the client's level. Watch for drowsiness, paresthesia, muscle twitching, convulsions, changes in mental status, and hypersensitivity reactions. Report increased levels and signs and symptoms of toxicity to physician.

REVIEW QUESTIONS
1. c   2. d   3. a   4. a   5. c   6. b   7. a   8. c
9. d   10. a

DYSRHYTHMIA ANALYSIS
1. Supraventricular tachycardia, adenosine (Adenocard)
2. Atrial fibrillation, digoxin (Lanoxin)
3. Sinus bradycardia, atropine
4. Premature ventricular contractions, lidocaine (Xylocaine)

Chapter 41

SHORT ANSWER
1. Atherosclerotic plaque in coronary arteries and coronary vasospasms
2. Atherosclerotic plaque narrows the lumen, decreases elasticity, and impairs dilation of coronary arteries, resulting in impaired blood flow to the myocardium

3. Classic, variant, and unstable
4. Substernal chest pain that is constricting, squeezing, or suffocating in nature. Radiates to jaw, neck, shoulder down the left or both arms or to back. Lasts about 5 minutes or less.
5. Organic nitrates, beta-adrenergic blocking agents, and calcium channel blocking agents

MATCHING
1. c   2. g   3. e   4. d   5. b   6. j   7. f   8. h
9. a   10. i

TRUE OR FALSE
1. f   2. t   3. f   4. t   5. f   6. t   7. f   8. t
9. f   10. t

CLINICAL CHALLENGE
Medication should not be chewed or crushed – may interfere with the sustained released action.

Reduces peripheral vascular resistance and concurrent use with the nitrate can quickly decrease blood pressure.

Avoid large meals, alcohol, smoking, and getting extremely cold. Take medication as directed, do not change dosage, and monitor for possible adverse effects.

REVIEW QUESTIONS
1. d   2. b   3. d   4. b   5. b   6. a   7. b   8. c
9. a   10. d

Chapter 42

MATCHING
1. a   2. e   3. b   4. d   5. c   6. f

FILL IN THE BLANK
1. adrenergic
2. dopamine
3. epinephrine
4. isoproterenol
5. metaraminol
6. norepinephrine (Levophed)
7. dobutamine, dopamine
8. norepinephrine
9. dobutamine
10. acidosis

CLINICAL CHALLENGE
Increased heart rate, myocardial contractility and blood pressure.

Adequate fluids are necessary for maximal pressor effect and to prevent acidosis, which decreases the effectiveness of the medication.

REVIEW QUESTIONS
1. c   2. a   3. b   4. c   5. b.   6. a   7. b   8. d
9. a   10. b

Chapter 43

TRUE OR FALSE
1. f   2. t   3. t   4. f   5. t   6. t   7. f   8. t
9. t   10. t

MATCHING
1. g   2. j   3. c   4. d   5. i   6. h   7. e   8. b
9. f   10. a

CLINICAL CHALLENGE
Between 0.5 and 10 mcg/kg/min

Decrease blood pressure

Check thiocyanate level. If level is more than 12 mg/dL, the medication should be stopped and another drug ordered.

REVIEW QUESTIONS
1. c   2. d   3. a   4. c   5. b   6. c   7. d   8. a
9. d   10. b

Chapter 44

FILL IN THE BLANK
1. volume, composition, pH
2. nephron
3. glomerulus, tubule
4. proximal tubule
5. edema

MATCHING
1. h   2. i   3. g   4. j   5. a   6. d   7. c
8. e   9. f   10. b

TRUE OR FALSE
1. f   2. f   3. t   4. t   5. f   6. t   7. t
8. t   9. t   10. t

CLINICAL CHALLENGE
Creatinine clearance level

Hearing loss

Take medication as prescribed, increase diet with foods high in potassium, decrease sodium intake, weigh daily

REVIEW QUESTIONS
1. c   2. b   3. a   4. a   5. a   6. c   7. b   8. d
9. b   10. a

THE NEPRON DIAGRAM
1. efferent arteriole
2. afferent arteriole
3. Bowman's capsule
4. glomerulus
5. distal tubule
6. proximal tubule
7. collecting tubule
8. descending limb of Henle's loop
9. ascending limb of Henle's loop
10. Henle's loop

Chapter 45

FILL IN THE BLANK
1. thrombosis
2. embolus
3. atherosclerosis
4. myocardial ischemia
5. homostasis

TRUE OR FALSE
1. t   2. f   3. f   4. t   5. f   6. t   7. t   8. f
9. t   10. f

FILL IN THE CHART

Drug	Increases	Decreases
acetaminophen	x	
griseofulvin		x
carbamazepine		x
tetracycline	x	
furosemide	x	
fluconazole	x	
rifampin		x
estrogen		x
aspirin	x	
quinidine	x	

CLINICAL CHALLENGE

Heparin helps prevent further thrombus formation and embolization.

Activated partial thromboplastin time will be done prior to administration of heparin and every 6 hours for 24 hours.

FILL IN THE CHART

Blood lipid	Desired level	Borderline level	High level
Triglycerides	<150 mg/dL	150–199 mg/dL	200 mg/dL
Total serum cholesterol	<200 mg/dL	200–239 mg/dL	240 mg/dL
LDL cholesterol	<100 mg/dL	130–159 mg/dL	160 mg/dL
HDL cholesterol	40–60 mg/dL	N/A	>60 mg/dL

TRUE OR FALSE

1. f   2. t   3. t   4. t   5. f   6. f   7. t   8. t
9. f   10. t

CLINICAL CHALLENGE

Assess his knowledge level about cholesterol, appropriate diet, foods he should avoid, etc. Discuss his weight, exercise, ask about support system at home. Explain adverse effects of flushing, pruritus. Encourage follow-up clinic visits to check cholesterol levels.
Can take ASA. Should take niacin with meals.

REVIEW QUESTIONS

1. a   2. a   3. c   4. b   5. d   6. a   7. b   8. c
9. b   10. b

Heparin does not dissolve the clots already formed. Bed rest will decrease risk of clots breaking off and traveling to the heart, lungs or brain. Monitor increased bleeding tendencies.

REVIEW QUESTIONS

1. b   2. c   3. c   4. b   5. a   6. b   7. b   8. d
9. b   10. a

Chapter 46

FILL IN THE BLANK

1. cholesterol, phospholipids, triglycerides
2. lipoproteins
3. serum
4. cholestyramine
5. lovastatin
6. fibrates
7. statin
8. gemfibrozil
9. fibrates, niacin
10. soy

Chapter 47

TRUE OR FALSE

1. f   2. t   3. t   4. t   5. f   6. f   7. t   8. f
9. t   10. t

FILL IN THE BLANK

1. stress
2. gastrin
3. aluminum, magnesium
4. bismuth
5. cimetidine
6. omeprazole (Prilosec)
7. misoprostol
8. sucralfate
9. omeprazole (Prilosec)
10. Mylanta, Maalox

MATCHING

1. d   2. a   3. h   4. c   5. i   6. g   7. e   8. j
9. b   10. f

CLINICAL CHALLENGE

To prevent the pumping or release of gastric acid from parietal cells into the stomach lumen and block the final step of acid production.

Nausea, diarrhea and headache

Between 4 and 8 weeks

Can be taken with or without food, swallow tablets, do not crush

REVIEW QUESTIONS

1. d   2. a   3. a   4. c   5. b   6. d   7. b   8. b
9. c   10. a

TRUE OR FALSE

1. t   2. t   3. f.   4. f   5. f   6. t   7. t   8. t
9. t   10. f

CLINICAL CHALLENGE

This drug antagonizes the receptors and prevents their activation by anticancer drugs, usually first-choice drugs.

Diarrhea, headache, dizziness, constipation, muscle aches

Dexamethasone (Decadron)

REVIEW QUESTIONS

1. a   2. b   3. c   4. b   5. a   6. d   7. d   8. b
9. b   10. c

Chapter 48

FILL IN THE BLANK

1. medulla oblongata
2. prochlorperazine (Compazine), promethazine (Phenergan)
3. benzodiazepines
4. dronabinol (Marinol)
5. meclizine (Antivert)
6. phosphorated carbohydrate solution (Emetrol)
7. scopolamine
8. metoclopramide (Reglan)
9. dolasetron (Anzemet)
10. dexamethasone (Decadron)